MASTER YOUR MIGRAINE

THE MIGRAINE HOME-CURE MANUAL

by

Ron H. Lange

with illustrations by
Jim Rhodes

Enigma Publishing

...contained in this book are not ...ith your physician. The reader ...natters relating to his or her health ...oms which may require diagnosis ...ng your health require medical supervision, and this book is not intended as a substitute for the medical advice of a physician.

The reader must recognize that the nature of care outlined in this book is such that it must be individualized.

The process to eradicate migraines described in this book is Patent Pending, and products developed for use in this process are Trademarked and held as Trade Secret and may not be used, nor may any products be manufactured for use in said process, by any entity either commercial or nonprofit without the written consent of the patent applicant, TM/TS holder. Permission for the use of this process is only granted herein to private individuals within the confines of their private lives and may not be administered to others for profit.

Copyright 1996 by Ron Lange
(Earlier non-published versions 1990–91)

First edition, February 1996
Library of Congress Number 95-083475
ISBN 0-9648931-0-X

Cover and illustrations by Jim Rhodes
Typography by Prototype, Albuquerque, NM

For additional copies of this book, send check or money order for $17.95 plus $4.00 shipping and handling per copy to:

Mail Service Department
Enigma Publishing Company
P.O. Box 75013
Albuquerque, NM 87194
Phone/FAX 899-3093

(Enigma Publishing cannot be responsible for cash sent in mail; discounts or partial refunds apply to additional copies.)

This lifelong effort is dedicated to my children

If it weren't for you, this effort may never have been undertaken. I desperately needed to give you and your descendents the ability to control a problem inherited from me. I love you.

CONTENTS

ACKNOWLEDGMENTS

Thanks to a higher power for the insight that stopped my suffering and allowed the intervention in the pain of others.

Thanks also to some special friends:

Tom Pierce, for encouraging me to start this work;

Elliott "Mike" Hendricks, for computerizing my original text, editing, and proofreading (Mike, what is a subjunctive anyway?);

Ed Thomas, fellow Trekkie, for proofreading and trying to get us on "Star Trek NG" (we would even have been Ferengie!);

Jim Rhodes, for illustrating this work with a God-given artistic talent;

Mary Ann Padilla, for helping with my tendency to be long-winded and wordy;

Michael Reed, for doing the editing that had been eluding us amateurs, and for bringing the project to fruition;

Lora McInnis, for inspiring the first effort to write. Instructions to her were my first attempt to put any of this on paper. We met while she remained in agony following a two-day hospital stay for a migraine. Later, I had the opportunity to eliminate her full-scale migraine in about twenty minutes, and she insisted on being the first to buy a manual that would be done in the future. Lora, I'm sorry it took five years.

INTRODUCTION

The pain started at a young age. A memory still persists of being about five and asking my father to give me a ride in the back seat of the family car so I could sleep and awaken without a headache. That was my first cure. I had once fallen asleep in the back seat with my head hurting while on a long drive and awoke to find the headache gone. It was quite specific though; it only worked with the combination of Dad's firm, safe "trucker grip" on the wheel, the snuggle of the huge back seat over a quietly rumbling exhaust, and the soft ride of the '49 Hudson.

I recall staring at the ceiling of the old farmhouse at age eleven, unable to move my eyes from pain. Other than prescription opiates there was really little that could be done, and in those days aspirin was the only pain reliever available. The migraine problem would also result in one being subjected to many indignities, from ice packs on the head to enemas.

As an adult, I realized that the migraine was a medical enigma. It seemed nothing could, or would, be done about it. I had children who stood to inherit this agony. Somewhere, I felt certain, a cure had to exist. Somewhere, there was another '49 Hudson.

It had to be simple. About one person in ten has this problem. I believed that since these people all have the same kind of headache, the headaches must all have the same cause—one singular cause. There is something within us that is universal, and it may not be complicated. But the world of western medicine seemed to think there was no solution to this dilemma. I began to think that maybe this is one of those times when a large group of people holds a false idea, like racism and prejudice, or catching a cold from cold air instead of a virus. The larger the group that holds the faulty belief, the more difficult it is to think your way against the tidal wave of communal conviction. But maybe, I thought, the more people who hold the belief and the higher the tide of public opinion, the higher the odds that they may all be wrong. With that in mind, I threw out all assumptions about migraines and started from nothing, not even taking for granted the idea that migraines originate in the head.

My theory for the singular origin of migraine development quickly evolved. The breakthrough was simple. As soon as the focus was off of the head, the cause became apparent. A simple malfunction was causing a normal chemical secretion to grow into a poison.

I then spent two decades experimenting and testing methods to control the process of migraine escalation. Once I understood the process, control was simple. Two things must be done. First, as a migraine sufferer you must learn what causes these headaches so you can stop giving them to yourself. Second, when a migraine starts you simply need to know how to clean up the toxic spill. The aspects of your lifestyle that may need to be changed, as well as methods to stop the migraine at all stages, are explained in detail. Feedback from a growing number of fellow sufferers suggests that the methods used to control a migraine are as universal as the headache itself.

For the record, any similarity to any other research or to anyone else's theory is purely coincidental, information from someone helped either directly or indirectly by information contained herein, or the commonality of truth. The process for controlling a migraine that is described in this book is patent pending.

A few other theories of migraine evolution and physiology are included in an attempt to give a perspective to the condition.

Read on, friends, migraines are a done deal!

MASTER YOUR MIGRAINE

I

Definition and Evolution

Our education in the art of living without the agony of migraines will begin by defining the specific headache that is the focus of this manual. The exact definition is important because some ambiguity exists as to which headache is actually called a migraine.

Part of the reason the definition is ambiguous is that the medical community is not in total agreement on the issue. This lack of conformity makes it difficult for the rest of us to have a clear-cut understanding of the problem.

Medical professionals have further confused the issue by misusing their own terms. An example of this problem is the term *cluster headaches*. This was originally used to describe headaches that occur in close succession. But at some point the term *cluster* was misinterpreted to mean some type of neuroelectrical storm or brain wave seizure, conjuring mental images of a painful attack, somewhat like epilepsy, that is confined to a small part of the brain. This error has led to examinations of brain waves, magnetic resonance images (MRIs), and computerized axial tomography (CAT) scans to look for these elusive storms in the brain. To compound this irony, these misguided exams are used regularly to confirm a migraine diagnosis. Figure that one out!

Another confusing term is *vascular headache*. The medical community refers to some migraines as "vascular" when the victim exhibits high blood pressure symptoms in the face, such as red eyes and a pink flush to the cheeks and ears. The truth is that all migraines are the same, but some sufferers are more prone to show red in the eyes and

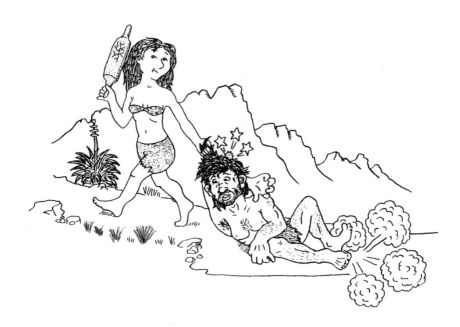

face. We all experience a profound pressure build-up in the upper back, the neck, and especially the head.

The lack of a proper definition has led us to this point: Most painful headaches are now generically referred to as "migraines." To clarify what is and what is not a migraine, this manual focuses on the most common type of extreme headache, the one most often called a migraine. (It is also referred to sometimes as the "sick headache".) This headache is characterized by extreme nausea and frequent vomiting. A more complete list of symptoms follows in the chapter titled Denial, Acceptance, and Early Detection. If you have ever had a headache that seemed to cause you to throw up, and especially if you then began a cycle of repetitive vomiting, you have had a migraine. You are one of the many victims.

Now that we can agree on which headache is actually a migraine, let's examine possible origins. We may even take a fleeting moment to appreciate them. That's right, appreciate them. If they are an evolved function, we may owe migraines a debt of gratitude, possibly for our very existence.

During aeons of evolution, our early ancestors were hunters and gatherers. Gathering very often amounted to scavenging. It is possible that the migraine phenomenon is a vestige of the early human condition that played a role in our survival. When our early ancestors managed to find more fresh food than they could eat, preserving it was not only difficult, it was often impossible. When excess food had spoiled, it was still eaten when hunger overpowered reason.

This problem was more common with the women. They were left with infants, small children, and a rotting food supply while the men were out foraging for more fresh food. The women were the last to eat the new-found meal, since the men would eat some of their bounty for the strength to return with their catch to the family. This well-known hunter scenario, and the fact that twice as many women as men have migraines, points to a possible evolutionary link.

This problem of eating spoiled food continued for millennia. There were only a few successes in the history of food storage. Civilizations by the sea learned to use salt as a preservative. The practice of drying sea water to harvest salt eventually led to mining. The discovery that salt could be dug from the ground facilitated the use of salt far from the sea, and its usage became widespread. People in arid climates who did not have salt nearby could only dry fresh meat, fruits, and vegetables for later consumption. Inhabitants of colder regions could pack food in snow or ice as long as they could manage to make it last.

These practices remained the state of the art for thousands of years. The most dramatic breakthrough in the history of food preservation occurred in the middle of the 19th century with the invention of canning. Contemporary civilization has only had the benefit of refrigeration since the 1920s. This is so recent that many people who saw the first mechanical refrigerators are still living today. Food storage methods that we now take for granted, such as freeze drying and vacuum packing, are literally space age developments; they have only been in commercial use since the era of space exploration. If the entire history of human evolution could be expressed in terms of a period of 24 hours, these modern advances would have occurred only within the last few seconds. For the previous 23 hours, 59 minutes, and 50-some seconds, our species would have had to cope with eating tainted, spoiled, and poisonous food.

Throughout human history the nausea and headache that we now call a migraine may have been a lifesaving mechanism that protected our forebears from food poisoning. The human digestive system inherited from its primate ancestors the ability to expel tainted food. I believe that the migraine sufferer's system may be the result of an evolutionary giant step beyond simply expelling food. Our digestive tracts may have taken a quantum leap in the ability to limit poisoned blood from reaching the brain. The migraine headache could be the

3

ultimate refinement in the art of expelling poisonous food, in the form of a cranial cramp.

This cramp would allow less blood to make contact with brain tissue by directly restricting the flow returning from the brain. This would account for the appearance of blood pressure build-up—the reddish color in the whites of the eyes and the pink flush to the face and ears. Other direct evidence also exists in extreme IQ declines during headaches that would result from decreased oxygen exposure to brain tissue. The physiological response that we call a migraine could have the ultimate purpose of preserving the brain during the presence of poison in the stomach, even if we create this poison within our own bodies.

If this picture of the evolutionary function of the migraine is accurate, it is a miraculous adaptation that has never been fully appreciated. But as important to human survival as the migraine may have been, it is now a function that has outlived its usefulness. In the day of modern food preservation, it is now as useless as the elusive purpose of the human appendix.

However migraines evolved, or whether they ever served a useful purpose, they are with us today in great abundance. Some conservative estimates suggest that one in five women and one out of ten men suffer from these headaches. More liberal calculations put the figure at over 50 percent of the world population. The latter view takes into account those who only suffer severe headaches on rare occasions. Regardless of which figures are more accurate, this is far too much suffering. Too many people have been in too much pain for far too long. Now that we have taken a moment to appreciate what migraines may have contributed to our species, let's move on and eradicate them.

II

The Migraine Process

*M*igraines are not in your head! Regardless of the amount of pain you may have experienced in your head, regardless of the number of doctors who have pondered your head, regardless of the amount of medication you have taken for your head, *migraines are not in your head!* They do not exist in your head psychologically, as figments of your imagination, nor are they produced by your subconscious, as many doctors believe. Most importantly, migraines are not in your head physically. They are not pains that start in your head because of some problem that exists there, as the majority of the medical community insists. The fact is, migraines result from a condition in your digestive tract which causes the pain in your head as a secondary reaction, a symptom, and there is nothing wrong with your head.

You probably feel that your headache is causing the nausea as the headache grows and you become increasingly sick to your stomach. This is the illusion that, until now, has always thwarted a cure. It has been impossible to develop a cure based on the physical cause when researchers were attempting to eliminate a symptom. In actuality, the opposite of this migraine illusion is true. The stomach acid started the headache in the beginning, long before you felt that the headache was causing the nausea.

The migraine machinery is set in motion by a food or circumstance that causes the stomach to secrete acids. An automatic reaction to the acid infusion is the closing of the "trap door" at the base of the stomach. This door is a muscular drawstring called the pyloric sphincter. It shuts any time acid is present to contain food for digestion. This is all quite normal and nothing has gone wrong—yet.

If you are a migraine sufferer, something else happens. Everyone has another chemical mix that is not designed to be in your stomach because it is not a stomach acid. This substance has the very limited purpose of breaking down food that has made it into the small intestine still intact. Its secretion is triggered by the presence of animal fat, cellulose fiber, nuts, sugar, and simply anything hard to digest. Unfortunately, it can even be secreted by tension, hunger, lack of sleep, or sometimes just because it's a certain time of the month. This culprit is bile, a mixture of chemicals that can make sulfuric acid (auto battery acid) when the bile contacts normal stomach acid.

A very simple thing happens to migraine victims: bile flows back into their stomachs. I don't know the mechanism by which bile finds its way into the stomach, but I suspect that the stomach sphincter is designed more to hold stuff in the stomach than to keep stuff out. It may be a kind of one-way valve. Regardless of how the bile gets in, it sure does, and you have seen it when you vomited during your headaches. I suspect that it simply flows back into the stomach because the arch of the duodenum is too high. This would cause people with smaller chest cavities, like women, to have more migraines than those with larger girths. The smaller chest width would contribute to a tighter

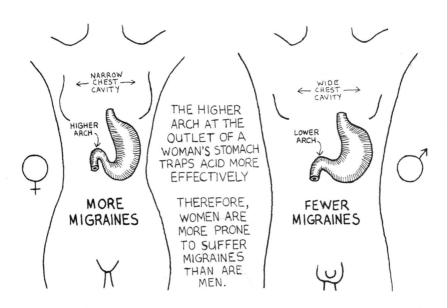

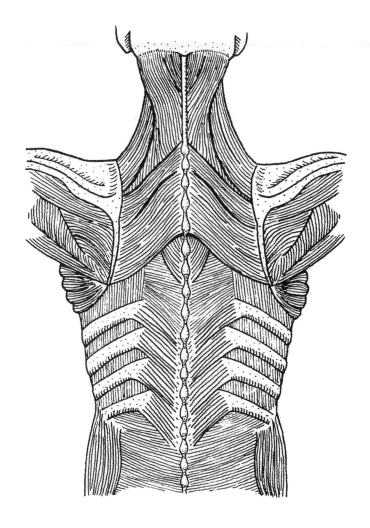

curvature at the beginning of the small intestine. The configuration of this intestinal shape would also be hereditary.

Now that chemical compounds found in your car battery are finding their way into your bloodstream, several reactions begin. First, the muscular structure, of which the stomach sphincter is an integral part, cramps to lock up the stomach and secure the poison for regurgitation. This set of connected muscle tissues extends from the middle of your back, up through your shoulder blades, and across your shoulders. The result of this cramp is a tightening discomfort in the middle of the back and shoulders. This shoulder ache then begins to include the neck and temples as the cramp tightens more profoundly. Now the headache has begun.

You move rapidly to the next level. It isn't just a headache anymore. You begin to feel nauseous as your stomach fills with acid to empty itself. It could end there: you throw up and it's over. But as you know, that's not what happens. Your system is confused by the concoction in the stomach and still believes that it must secrete bile. The bile is still somehow sliding through the closed sphincter into the stomach. The stomach still senses a poison and continues to infuse any liquid that it can muster in the attempt to flush it out. The event has become cyclical. Later in the book we will refer to this as "cyclical acid poisoning" or CAP.

Now your headache moves on to another level. The toxic chemical spill in your stomach is truly beginning to poison you. What started as simple nausea is now "sickness" beyond description. You no longer simply have a headache; your head pain has skyrocketed as the muscles around the neck, the back of the head, the temples, and behind the eyes cramp to slow the poisoned blood's contact with your brain tissue. There is no way to describe this level of sickness to someone who doesn't have migraines. You feel that death is imminent. But this has happened before, and you know you won't be that lucky.

DETAILED DESCRIPTION OF A MIGRAINE'S DEVELOPMENT

- The stomach's sensing nerves detect either a substance that is not digestible by ordinary stomach acid or certain conditions such as tension, causing the backup digestive system to respond by secreting bile into the duodenum.
- The bile goes the wrong way and enters the stomach through the back door. At the detection of the wrong acid in the stomach, the sensing nerves secrete still more acid as their only possible response.
- The sensors detect an acid overload, and the body's protective system is set into motion. The brain sends a signal to the muscular structure that includes the sphincter at the base of the stomach. It reacts by cramping. This closes off the continuation of the digestive tract into the small intestine.
- The stomach fills with normal acids and other liquids that the body scavenges from other organs to purge itself of a foreign chemical.
- The bloodstream becomes poisoned. Normal acids cannot enter the bloodstream because the stomach lining filters them out. But bile is not designed for the stomach, and the lining is not developed to filter out its caustic chemical components.
- The stomach continues to fill until the gag response takes over to purge the acid. After emptying, there is some relief until the stomach

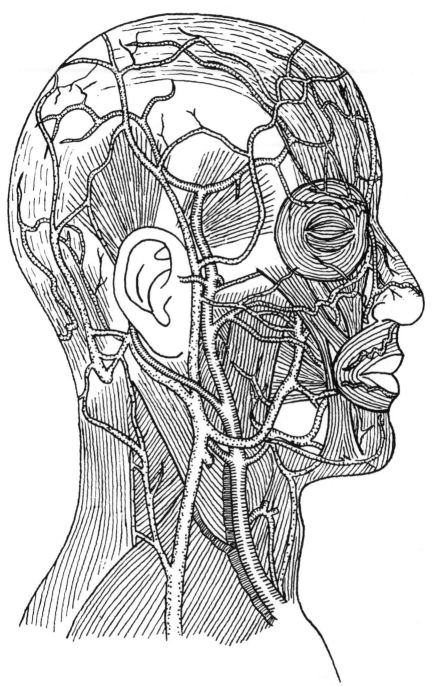

THE MUSCULAR STRUCTURE THAT CRAMPS TO SLOW BLOOD FLOW

9

can refill again. It will refill because the bile mechanism is still sensing excess acid in the stomach, which still indicates the presence of something indigestible. Meanwhile, the stomach is continuing to infuse acid because it is sensing the presence of bile. The normal acid stimulates bile, which enters the stomach and in turn stimulates more acid . . . more bile . . . more acid . . . ad infinitum.

• The headache has now become cyclical. This self-perpetuating nature is fundamental to a migraine. If it isn't cyclical, it isn't a migraine. The CAP can continue for days, with extreme misery and other real health concerns due to dehydration from rapid liquid loss.

• As the brain sends a signal to the stomach sphincter to cramp and lock up, all of the muscles along the upper spine, through the back of the neck, and around the skull also cramp. The cranial cramp is the headache. This cramp is designed to restrict the blood flow and slow its passage through brain tissue until the poison is no longer present. This restriction causes blood pressure to build up in the head, with the sensation that your head is ready to explode.

• You are now trapped in the CAP effect and feel hopelessly overwhelmed by a poisoned delirium. Within this hellish existence is a world of extreme nausea, tightening of the upper back and neck, and unrelenting head pain. There is no way to break out of the poisoning cycle. No nutrition can reach the bloodstream because any food eaten to provide nutrition will be expelled by a gag response to the acid produced.

III

Learning to Prevent Migraines

The most important migraine treatment strategy is to learn to avoid them. It is far easier not to allow the spark of a headache to ignite than to manage the raging inferno of a migraine. Later in the manual you will see how to treat the inferno, but for now let's look at avoiding the spark.

"Forewarned is forearmed." This old adage is aptly applied to migraines, and it is the first rule in mastering them. Understanding the workings of migraine mechanics is the first tool necessary for living without this agony. The second tool is an instinctive understanding of the things that will set those mechanisms in motion.

You must first learn your triggers! These are foods, drinks, or occurrences that will activate your migraine. Many triggers are universal among sufferers, and the following list contains the most common culprits. At the end of this book a page has been added for your own notes. You may want to include all the special foods, beverages, and circumstances that set you up for a migraine.

COMMON TRIGGERS AND SUGGESTED EDIBLE AMOUNTS

1. *Animal fat*.
   • *Fatty meats*, such as hot dogs, sausage, cold cuts, and hamburger, are devastating triggers. The amount you can eat depends on the meat, the amount of fat, and how it's cooked. Very fatty meats can be boiled or broiled to lessen fat content. Use common sense when eating meat heavy with fat. Cut off as much fat as you can, cook

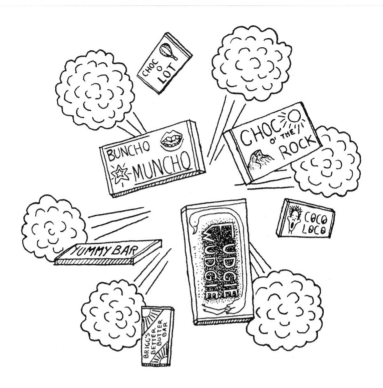

out as much grease as possible, and eat only small amounts (2–3 oz).

• *Roast beef* appears more innocent than it really is, because the fat cooks into the meat. Eat only small amounts (2–3 oz).

• *Steak* is normally grilled, so the fat is not cooked into the meat as much as with roast beef. Eat moderate amounts (4–5 oz).

• *Cheese* is the single worst trigger. Eat very small amounts (½ oz) unless it is low-fat cheese (such as mozzarella); then more (1 oz) can be eaten. Now that non-fat cheese has finally appeared on the market, you can have more (2 oz), but you must still exercise caution. Even with fat-free products, some of the molecules that stimulate acid production are present.

• *Whole milk* will give you an instant migraine. The less fat the milk has, the more you may have. Skim milk has very little triggering effect.

• *Ice cream* is terrible; you may as well sit down with a spoon and a tub of lard. You could get away with eating a little low-fat ice cream (3–4 oz). Ice milk is better (4–5 oz), but you must keep an eye on the labeled fat content. Making it at home with skim milk is best, but no dairy company that I know of makes skim ice milk. They do make no-fat now, and if it weren't too sweet, you could have about all of it you wanted. Unfortunately, everything I've tried (and I love ice cream) has been too sweet. Someday, someone will get it right.

2. *Sugar* is a trigger if very concentrated, such as in frosting, candy, and candy bars. Eat very small amounts (½ oz).

3. *Chocolate* has tropical oil–type fat and concentrated sugar, both of which are triggers. Eat very small amounts (½ oz).

4. *Peanut butter* contains peanut oil (also used in Oriental cooking), which is particularly troublesome. Eat very small amounts (½ oz).

5. *Nuts* have a high oil content with a structure similar to peanut oil and also need acid to break up the solid, unchewed kernels. Eat only small amounts (1 oz).

6. *Sunflower seeds* are an instant trigger. Eat none.

7. *Undercooked beans*, such as pork and beans or other canned beans, are not fully cooked for canning and require stomach acid to break them down. Eat none, they are an instant trigger. If the beans are cooked longer to remove the crunch, they have no triggering effect.

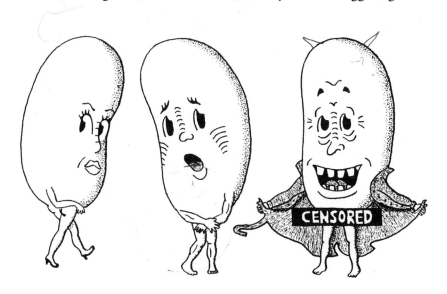

RAW BEANS

13

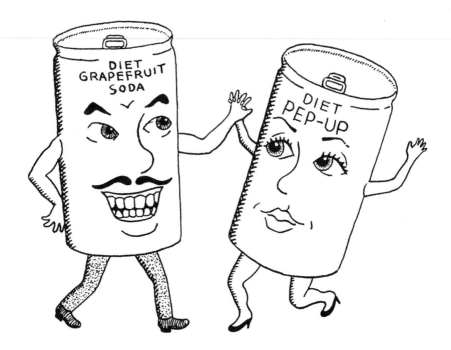

8. *Some artificially sweetened sodas* are instant triggers. This is very subjective, and you will have to try most sodas on an individual basis. It may be entirely personal, but Diet Squirt and Diet Dr Pepper are instant triggers for me. I can drink only 6 oz of either. Until you know how much you can consume of any artificially sweetened drink, be cautious. Later we will look at artificial sweeteners in more detail, because they have both positive and negative effects.

9. *Alcoholic beverages* are pretty much on the no-can-do list because we sufferers must use pain relievers that are hard on either our livers or our stomachs. Alcohol is harmful to both, multiplying the danger and the effect of the damage. But some of us are going to drink a little anyway, so let's examine alcohol's impact on the migraine.

    For the sufferer, alcohol produces three different headaches:

    • A migraine can start immediately from residual by-products in the beverage as soon as only a small amount is consumed. Beer and wine are more damaging than other beverages in this regard. This is another instance that must be considered on a personal level. Some brands have little effect, while others are devastating.

    • As the liver attempts to process the alcohol, a hangover will develop from any type of alcohol consumed. At this point the hangover is not yet a migraine.

    • For the migraine victim, the hangover will develop into a full-

14

scale, devastating migraine. The cure described later in the manual does not work as quickly or as well on a hangover as it does on a migraine. The successes that have been observed are difficult to analyze, because it is impossible to know where you are between the hangover and the migraine. But when all the residual hangover-causing agents have been cleaned out by the liver and the hangover has become locked into a migraine, the cure works as well as with any other migraine. This depends entirely on how well the alcohol has been removed from the blood. At what point the hangover becomes a migraine is a very gray area, and the only approach is to start working on the headache while it is still in the hangover stage. To handle this, refer to the chapter titled Curing the Migraine Before It Starts.

CAUTION: Recent information has shown acetaminophen to cause liver damage when used with alcohol. I suggest using only ibuprofen following the ingestion of any alcohol, and even with ibuprofen it may be wise to limit the amount you take to half your normal dosage.

HANGOVER/MIGRAINE ADVICE: Naturally, migraine sufferers are best served by not drinking. But if you're going to drink anyway, and you promise not to drive, I'll give you a pointer. If you drink mixed drinks with either a citric base (e.g., Collins mix, Margarita mix, grapefruit soda, orange juice, and grapefruit juice) or with a tomato juice base, you may escape migraine free. This will become clearer after further reading.

10. *Tea, hot or iced*, is a trigger due to tannic acid. Hot tea can be buffered with milk or creamer to offset its triggering response. Iced tea is one of the most overlooked triggers and can only be consumed in small amounts (6 oz).

11. *Coffee, black*, contains an acrid oil that will start a headache if not buffered with milk or creamer.

12. *Highly acidic or sweet juices* overstimulate the stomach sensors and trigger acid production.

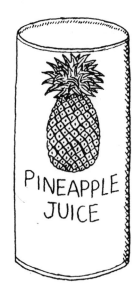

• *Pineapple juice* is too sweet. Drink none, and eat only small amounts of the fruit (4 oz).

• *Grapefruit juice* is too acidic. Drink small amounts (4 oz), and eat only moderate amounts of the fruit (½ a whole fruit).

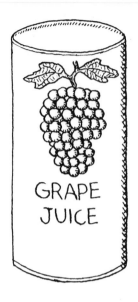
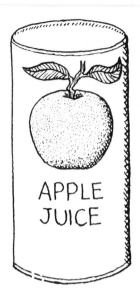
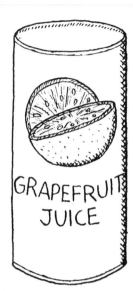

GRAPE
JUICE

APPLE
JUICE

GRAPEFRUIT
JUICE

- *Apple juice* is too concentrated, and therefore too sweet. Drink only small amounts (4 oz), but eat all the fruit you want.
- *Grape juice* is also too concentrated and too sweet. Drink small amounts (4 oz), and eat only moderate amounts (6–8 oz) of the fruit.
- *V8 juice* has ingredients other than tomato juice which make it a trigger. Just don't drink it, even if it is a "zippy sort of thing." This does not apply to tomato juice, which is a very beneficial drink (discussed later).

13. *Watermelon* is especially bad. Eat small amounts (4–6 oz). Cantaloupe, muskmelons, and honeydew are triggers only if a lot is eaten.

14. *Lettuce and other hard-to-digest raw vegetables* will really get your bad juices flowing. Lettuce is the worst because you are forced to eat more of it. It's everywhere, in everything, and in terms of digestibility, you may as well eat your lawn. Eat very small amounts, only one leaf on a sandwich or a couple bites of a dinner salad. You can get away with most other raw vegetables, but limit yourself to 4 oz.

15. *Bell pepper* is another particularly bad vegetable. You should avoid it raw and in the dreaded stuffed bell pepper. You can survive it cooked if you only eat small amounts, but when you eat one or two whole peppers and add greasy meat, you're in for trouble. Bell peppers are the only pod pepper that I know of (and I'm a chile addict), regardless of the hotness factor, with a triggering

16

effect. As a side note, most other chile pod types have a beneficial effect. Pepper pod dishes have been used in the Hispanic culture for centuries to solve stomach-related problems as well as headaches and hangovers. A green chile stew is excellent to eat after you have eliminated your headache, not to mention after you've had too much tequila. Hispanic people often move straight from tequila to menudo without passing Go. I don't advise it. They're tougher folks than most of us. But I've been told either green chile or menudo will stop even the hangover.

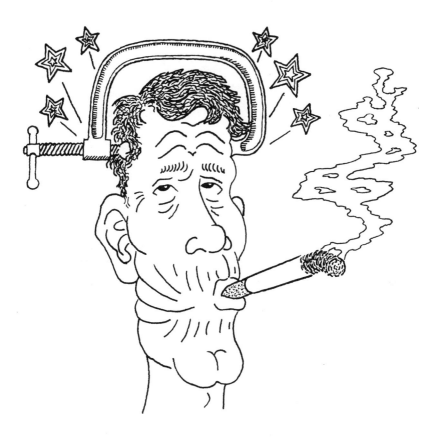

16. *Tobacco smoke* can start the headache but is especially bad if a headache has already begun. Secondary smoke is intolerable and will instantly make your migraine worse, even at a considerable distance from the smoker. Nicotine causes capillaries to restrict, and vascular restriction is fundamental to a headache. Nicotine dramatically enhances this process.

17. *Oriental food* has a surprisingly bad effect. The basic ingredients are healthy, nutritious, and beneficial foods for migraine-free meals. Unfortunately, most restaurants use monosodium glutamate (MSG) and peanut oil, both of which are triggers.
18. *Vitamins* on an empty stomach will start a headache. Heavy doses will start one too, even if you have food in your stomach. The oil-based ones like A, D, E and K are especially bad unless you take them with food.
19. *Tension* is easily the next largest cause of migraines, after food. There is an endless list of special circumstances that can cause tension and set the migraine process in motion. Pressure from your job, being caught in traffic, marital and monetary problems are just a few examples. Any situation that causes stress or tension can start the CAP response. Some highly sensitive people can set the migraine machinery in motion simply by sitting or lying in an uncomfortable position. The ultimate in migraine sensitivity is to have one triggered by looking at a bright light or smelling an unpleasant aroma.

This list is a very basic guide to give you a start on visualizing your triggers. The possible ways to begin the cyclical gastric secretion and subsequent poisoning are as varied and numerous as we migraine sufferers of the world. This is why each victim must pay close attention to his or her own special migraine triggers. There are a few other categories of triggers, such as lack of sleep, overeating, and getting too hungry, which we will discuss later in separate chapters.

IV

Trigger Combinations

Combining migraine triggers is especially dangerous and difficult to avoid. For example, a dinner as apparently innocent as roast beef, mashed potatoes made with whole milk and butter, gravy, a glass of whole milk, and a scoop of ice cream for dessert is a virtual migraine cocktail. The only item listed that will not give you a migraine is the potatoes. Even those innocent spuds have included the two triggers of butter and milk, and a third is added when you top them with gravy. This meal has six triggers; the average migraine victim won't make it through the night unscathed. Equally bad are meals smothered with cheese, such as Italian or Mexican food, especially if accompanied by other triggers like whole milk, iced tea, or ice cream.

The danger of multiple triggers is the number one problem with migraines. You may know to stay away from milk and cheese at the same meal, but you may slip up and have iced tea. Many other combinations are equally threatening; the list is endless. Refer to the trigger list when you are planning a meal or even a light late-night snack. Once again, remember to expand this list to include your own special migraine triggers.

While we're on the subject, let's not fly by that late-night snack without a warning. The late snack is particularly dangerous because you will be going to bed and becoming unconscious shortly after eating it. You must take extra caution not to eat any triggers at this time. The problem is that the migraine will develop while you are asleep. This is such an immense problem for victims that we will address it later in

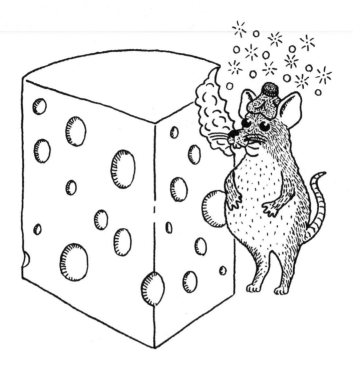

a chapter dedicated solely to this singular phenomenon.

Most sufferers respond to all of the listed common triggers and to an extensive personal list as well. Some people have had their lives incapacitated by the number of triggers that will put them into a migraine delirium. Taking into view the number of possible trigger combinations, you can easily see how this problem can escalate into a very bad day.

The danger of trigger combinations makes it critical that you memorize all of the common triggers and all of your personal ones. It's not so hard to do; there is a shorthand method of recalling these culprit foods that will remove a large portion of the memorization. About 75 percent of your headaches are started by one common ingredient: animal fat. In the roast beef dinner listed above, every item was a trigger, but animal fat was actually the only triggering substance involved. All you need to know is:

- watch for animal fat;
- memorize the few remaining common triggers;
- be aware of your personal triggers, which you have already learned the hard way.

It will not be necessary to concern yourself with the enormous number of possible combinations. When you see a known trigger in a meal, an automatic mental warning flag will go up. The more triggers in a meal, the more flags, and the more caution you will instinctively take. This will become as easy and natural as any other everyday activity. Handling the negative combinations will automatically fall into place as you begin to recognize your triggers.

V

Tricks for Triggers

D o not be distressed! You can eat your favorite foods in moderation, even though they are headache triggers. This is done by using positive or favorable combinations of foods. The object of a positive food combination is to have a food or drink with your meal that will *trick* your stomach out of secreting excess acid. This is an essential tool and is as important as knowing your triggers. *Learn what foods work to offset your acidic system, just as you have learned what foods will trigger it.*

The principle in tricking your stomach out of the migraine response is simply to give your system a food or drink with a *healthy acidity*. This is an acidity that is neither too strong nor too sweet. There are foods, and especially some drinks, that cause the stomach sensors to detect an optimal acidity level and allow consumption of other foods that are normally migraine triggers.

A good example of the perfect drink with any meal is unsweetened orange juice. To the migraine sufferer a nonsweet, mildly acidic drink is a miracle drug. It allows you to consume a meal that includes triggers without having a negative response. There are several other foods and beverages that work similarly.

The principle is the one used by the proverbial pregnant woman who craves pickles and ice cream. She has apparently spent considerable time in the throes of morning sickness, or possibly nature has endowed her with an instinctive understanding of combining food. She knows that if she eats a pickle (a migraine trick), she can then eat the ice cream (a migraine trigger) and trick her stomach out of secreting an acidic flow and starting a nausea response. Her stomach will sense the pickle's acidity and allow her to enjoy the ice cream, without nausea, in veritable pregnant bliss.

Nature has equipped pregnant women with finely tuned instincts for food combination and consumption. The "pickle and ice cream" approach is the concept that migraine sufferers must learn and practice in order to lead a normal life. The pickle trick uses the same principle as the orange juice trick. Having any form of tart pickle (dill, sour, Polish, kosher, etc.) or its juice with a meal is a healthy way to offset a sufferer's own acidity.

It is important to be aware that some fruits and juices are too acidic and/or too sweet. These are migraine triggers which will start your gastric juice flowing as a reaction and work against you instead of for you. Avoid using anything listed in the section on triggers, and most of all use your common sense.

SOME MILDLY ACIDIC DRINKS AND FOODS TO HAVE WITH MEALS

1. *Orange juice*, unsweetened, is the best trick of all.
2. *Citric drinks*, such as lemonade, limeade, and lemon-lime combinations, are very good if not too sweet. The powdered citric drinks work as well at fooling the stomach. Those with aspartame (Nutrasweet) work even better. They allow a very low sugar content, thus removing any sweetness-related trigger response. There are certain instances when a sweetener is an asset to the sufferer and other instances when it becomes a detriment. We need to pause here for a quick look at sweeteners.

   Saccharin is generally a trigger, so simply avoid it. Aspartame is only a trigger if you consume more than two packets of Equal or two sodas with Nutrasweet. As long as you use less aspartame than this within a two-hour period, it is beneficial since it replaces sugar. It is especially beneficial in citric drinks because the mild acidity offsets any trigger response. Naturally, this is recommended with the understanding that you do not have any allergies to artificial sweeteners.
3. *Combination citric drinks*, like the frozen concentrates in the freezer section at the grocery with several types of fruit juices included in them, are good if they do not have the wrong types of juices or have added sugar. Sweetness is very subjective, but in general, if you get the impression that the drink is sweeter than it is citric, you are probably drinking a trigger. Avoid juices that contain apple, grape, pineapple, and papaya. They are all too sweet.
4. *Grapefruit sodas*, like Squirt (*not* diet, mentioned in Triggers), are

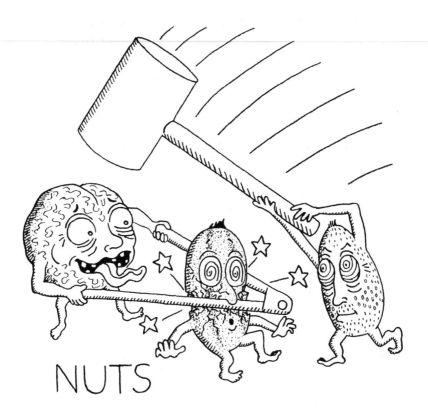

NUTS

good. Regular grapefruit soda is an excellent tricker.

5. *Tomato juice* works well, but stay away from tomato-based juices which are triggers because of other additives (such as V8 juice).

6. *Pickle juice* works great. Some may think you are a little on the fringe for drinking some with a meal, but it tastes exactly like the pickle that comes in it and offsets a migraine response beautifully.

7. *Cranberry juice* works too, but must have very little added sugar.

8. *Ketchup* can be used to smother everything. Now you can put it on your steak in a fancy restaurant and still be chic.

9. *Fruits and vegetables* are excellent for the most part, even though the processed juice from that fruit or vegetable may be a trigger. Fresh apples are a good example of this. In juice form they are too concentrated and too sweet. On the other hand, the actual fruit is perfect in sugar and acidity levels. Even a grapefruit is good to eat for the right acidity level to offset greasy food if you eat only half a fruit at a meal.

The following are absorbents that work by using the acidity to break down starch into complex carbohydrates and neutralize the acid in the process. This process is discussed in more detail later in the manual.

10. *Breads* are very good to eat if not heavy with fat, sweets, nuts, or sunflower seeds. Consume pastries sparingly. Most sweetbreads are heavily larded, overly sweetened, and contain nuts.

11. *Potatoes* are great any way they are cooked other than fried in animal fat. The only difficulty with potatoes is what you put on them. Most animal fat–based gravies will cause a migraine. The intrinsic problem with most gravy is that, even if all the fat or grease is drained from the meat broth, the process of cooking the meat homogenizes the fat into the water. Fat can exist unseen, much as cream is whipped into milk to make whole milk. Butter and sour cream are also triggers that need to be consumed in small amounts. French fries are very good if fried in hot vegetable oil (especially Canola) but bad if fried soggy at a low temperature or in animal fat. When using fries as a tricking mechanism, you can throw on all the ketchup you like. That's the way you like them anyway, isn't it?

12. *Pastas* are very good, but eat them with tomato sauce and use cream sauce and cheese sparingly.

Most foods that cause migraines are fatty, contain cholesterol, or are excessively sweet or overly acidic. They also often contain unhealthy chemicals, such as artificial sweeteners, MSG, or nitrates. Foods that are not migraine triggers are usually very healthy and natural. Learning to consume non-triggering foods will pay off in more ways than mere migraine avoidance. There will be the dividend of improvement in overall health. People who have followed these guidelines have also experienced significant weight loss.

EXCESS ACIDITY WARNING

Some sufferers who have read this section on using mild, unsweetened acidity to replace their own stomach acid have made a harmful assumption. If it makes sense to replace the acid during a meal that includes trigger foods, then doesn't it also make sense to drink a mildly acidic drink continually and replace the acid indefinitely? Can't we replace our acid permanently and never suffer from migraines again?

Unfortunately, there is a problem with using this method to achieve a headache-free life. You can overdose on acidity and cause other health problems to arise. A secondary problem for us migraine sufferers is over-supplying our body's store of acid.

In one case in which this method was tried, the individual drank orange juice continuously with good success in the beginning. Then the headaches returned with a vengeance. It appears that the body may

25

take elements from acidic food and drink to convert and store as its own gastric acid supply. In consuming an unnatural amount of acid, you could sabotage yourself by storing more acid than normal, which may become a problem later. This will eventually result in more migraines, more easily triggered and more often.

There is a quote attributed to Mae West, "If some's good, more's better." In the case of acidic drink, an old adage is more appropriate: "Moderation in everything, except stuff you really like."

Okay, maybe that's a new adage.

VI

A Few Tips on Cooking

In most instances the migraine machinery is set in motion by the body's need to break down something in the stomach. Food preparation can assist in averting this process by requiring the stomach to produce less acid. The removal of fat from meats before and after cooking is the most important step you can take.

For a good example of how to cook a fatty meat product, let's look at ground beef. It is one of the fattiest and most commonly used meat products. If you are preparing a meal based on fried ground beef, start by purchasing the leanest hamburger available. After frying a beef patty, drain it well and blot it with a paper towel. This method of fat removal should also be used on other fatty meats, such as bacon, sausage, and ham. If you are frying loose hamburger, put the meat in a strainer after it is cooked and run hot water through it to remove the grease.

When boiling meats like roast beef, stew meat, or chicken, skim the oil off the top after cooking. Set the pot away from the heat for a few minutes to allow the oil to surface. If the meat you are cooking is very fat laden, like cheaper cuts of roast or Polish sausage, even after taking these precautions you should only eat small portions (3–4 oz). Be careful with the amount of broth that you consume from a high-fat meat source (1–2 oz). The simple rules are: *When you see grease, blot it up, wash it out, or skim it off.* And remember: *If there was a lot of fat in the meat, don't eat a lot of the gravy.*

Grandma's ''fryin's gravy'' is another type of gravy made from an even more fat-laden source. I recall as a child seeing gravy being made

27

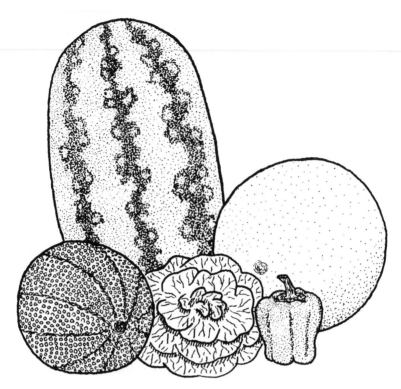

MELONS, LETTUCE, & BELL PEPPER TRIGGERS

from fried meat, especially chicken, by combining grease, fryings, and flour into a paste and then heating and thinning it with either milk or water. The migraine experience has taught me a vital lesson in cooking: *Never use the grease from anything to make gravy.* Gravy is such a migraine trap that I use a simple method to eliminate the triggering effect. I just heat fat-free broth, season, and thicken with corn starch.

Some foods must be well cooked or they will cause an excess of acid production. Meats generally fall into this category, but there are other foods that do too. All types of beans must be cooked well beyond the feel of a crunch when chewed. Remember that beans from a can are still crunchy because canning companies want their products to remain firm until they are used by the consumer. The canned beans can then be reheated without becoming overcooked.

Another problem in the area of cooking is knowing which vegetables need to be cooked, which do not, and which are somewhere in between. Several fresh vegetables are considered chic when blanched, which causes them to fall into a vague area. Use this rule of thumb: *Any vegetable that you can eat raw without a triggering effect can also be eaten blanched.* Some vegetables, such as lettuce, can only be eaten in small

28

amounts raw, and you probably wouldn't like them much cooked, either (yuck!). Also remember that you can get a headache from almost any raw vegetable, such as carrots or celery, if you eat more than 4 oz at one meal.

Examples such as these must be considered on an individual basis, because personal responses vary. All of these variables and personalized instances may be somewhat overwhelming, but there is an easy way to handle any vegetable that may be in question. From a migraine standpoint, eat only small amounts of raw veggies, very little lettuce, no bell pepper, and cook the heck out of anything else.

I hope these few examples of cooking techniques will help you develop a basic concept of food preparation and assist you in living a migraine-free life. By keeping a focus on the food you eat and how it is prepared, you will stop many headaches before they start. As always, you must remember your own special circumstances in the fine art of migraine-free food selection and preparation.

VII

Denial, Acceptance, and Early Detection

It is very important to learn to recognize a migraine in its infancy, when it is only an average headache and can be treated with ordinary measures. Then you must act on it immediately.

Denial is a major problem you may have experienced in recognizing a headache early. The lack of a cure has made denial a tool that you have been forced to use. You may have attempted to ignore an approaching headache in the hope that it will not develop into a migraine. Or you may have felt that by relaxing and not thinking about it, the headache would not continue to grow. This technique is actually encouraged by medical practitioners and will work to a limited degree on a normal tension headache. But it won't work on a migraine. To deny that one is starting only allows it to grow and makes the cleanup process longer and more involved. Invariably you will experience discomfort longer and more profoundly.

To notice the oncoming headache before it becomes a full-scale migraine is the most important tool you can use to shorten the length of time necessary for a cure to work. Without denial you can accept the early symptoms and address them quickly.

A full understanding of all causes, the mechanics of the process, and the knowledge of a cure allow a positive approach to your symptoms. With this understanding, you can relax without the panic and fear that only aggravate a headache. Knowing that a cure is simple and easy will allow you to welcome the earliest symptoms and approach them aggressively, without the usual anxiety. First, get to know your early symptoms. Next, learn how to respond with the information you are learning. Then, when the next one makes its unwelcome visit, simply accept it, take action, and handle it . . . *you have it mastered.*

DETECT SYMPTOMS EARLY

Most early symptoms are universal. They may differ from yours, but in general they include:
- tightening in the temples;
- pressure in and behind the eyes;
- lack of vision, or spots in the vision;
- tension in the muscles along the upper spine between the shoulder blades;
- tension and ache in the back of the neck;
- tension and ache up the back of the head and behind the ears on the mastoid bone;
- nausea;
- reddening in the whites of the eyes, and;
- your own special early warning system symptom(s). A lifetime of experience with the onset of migraines may have armed you with your own personal early-detection device. I have a very slight clicking sound in the back of my neck, right at the base of my skull. It gives me the feeling that a ratchet is being used to tighten the muscles. You may have a sensation so slight that it prompts the feeling of "just knowing" a migraine is coming. Do not ignore this early warning, which may be unique to you—it is your best friend.

VIII

The Early Migraine Cure

N ow that you have learned to detect the earliest nuances of an
approaching headache, there are ways to stop most migraines
before they become a problem. This is the point at which you must
start to control your headache. There will be times that too many
triggers have been ingested and you simply cannot stop the migraine's
escalation. So I will show you how to approach the early cure with
the understanding that you may have to follow up immediately with
the full cure.

The method used to cure the early-stage migraine can also be applied to the average headache, but with migraines you must remember
the tricks and triggers aspects that further complicate the cleanup. For
example, you wouldn't want to take a pain reliever with a trigger drink
like whole milk to swallow the tablets. With that in mind, let's take
a look at stopping a migraine as it starts. Later we will build on the
early-cure information to learn how to eliminate a full-scale migraine.

The early-stage migraine is similar in severity to a normal headache.
The only real difference is that migraine sufferers know from experience
that the present pain is only the beginning. Although the migraine
starts as an average headache, it will continue to a higher level of inten-
sity as it becomes compounded by nausea.

As we know, headaches are cramps. In the early cure you can easily
unlock these cramping muscles. The cyclical acid poisoning (CAP)
factor is not fully established, and the stomach is not yet full of acid.
You can unlock the cramp of the sphincter at the base of the stomach

as you also ease the cramps in the back, neck, and cranial muscles. ⸀ unlocked sphincter allows anything in the stomach to empty into small intestine and stops the headache escalation.

To unlock the cramping sphincter, two problems must be addressed. This is true with both the early-symptom cure and the full-scale migraine cure.

PROBLEM #1: The stomach's acidity-sensing nerves must detect a drop in the amount of gastric acid present. This is important to catch early, because the acid will soon start the CAP effect. The solution: Neutralize the acidity with any good antacid, such as Mylanta, Riapan, Maalox, Digel, or baking soda. Regardless of how you neutralize your gastric juices, your acidity level is lowered and problem number one is solved. The sensors can quit calling in additional acid to help rid the previous stomach acid.

PROBLEM #2: To further prevent the acid from "bottling," the brain must fully release the lock at the base of the stomach. Along with the brain sensing a drop in acidity, it must also sense a decrease in pain. Pain causes a continued lock, even if the pH level is totally neutralized or the acid is expelled. The solution: A pain reliever must be taken two or three minutes after the antacid so that the brain can detect both changes. You need to wait a few minutes to let neutralization occur before throwing in more chemicals.

There is an interesting point about pain. It seems to take on a life of its own at an early point in the headache process. When that pain becomes "locked in," only a pain reliever can derail the pain-locking process. In a way, the pain reliever plays a trick on the brain. By artificially lowering the pain level, the drug tells the brain that the problem it has been experiencing is now over and it can relax its hold on the muscular structure. There are actually two locking mechanisms involved: the pain lock, which functions at a subconscious level; and the muscular structure cramp, which includes the stomach sphincter lock.

Anyone who has ever gone to a doctor with a migraine knows that there are no pain relievers, short of pure morphine, that will stop one. Physicians can inject you with Demerol or prescribe Darvon or codeine. The list is endless, but nothing stops the pain entirely without side effects. Most of these drugs don't really stop the headache; they simply put you into a delirium where you don't really care that you hurt. The drugs normally prescribed usually alter your perception or have other negative consequences. The very latest oral drug on the market reportedly has only a 70 percent success rate and has side effects. The FDA has approved a self injection that still causes a drugged feeling. This tells me that once again only the symptoms are being treated.

On the other hand, knowledge can replace the needle, the suffering, doctors' fees, drug expenses, and having to beg someone else for your relief. The cure in this manual uses common products that can be purchased at any grocery store. We use them in a new way to remove the pain and nausea at their source.

After the brain has detected an acidity drop, there are two familiar over-the-counter (OTC) products which will open the stomach sphincter while they diminish the pain. *The stomach will then empty into the small intestine. After the poisoning substance has been removed, the remainder of the headache and any ensuing nausea will disappear.*

Two familiar OTC products, acetaminophen (Tylenol) and ibuprofen (Advil), will usually work on the early migraine as well as they do on the average headache. To some extent their success is due to relaxing a cramp and opening the stomach. These products deserve more credit than we ever give them. Just imagine life without them! I have been reluctant to use aspirin, because migraines require heavy doses that may thin the blood too much and damage stomach lining. However, acetaminophen and ibuprofen are relatively safe and become true miracle drugs when used to assist in a migraine cure. Fortunately for us all, we can find them at our corner convenience store, and we don't have to pay anyone for permission to use them.

A large part of their success with migraines lies in taking a strong enough dose to power through the pain sufficiently to open the stomach. This involves using the proper medication, at an adequate dosage, for the right degree of a headache. The proper dosage with previous acid neutralization adds extra effectiveness. An important step in using these two common pain relievers is to take another look at the recommended doses on their containers. We migraine sufferers need a precise way to determine an effective amount that still remains safe.

Throughout the many years that acetaminophen has been available OTC to the public, it has always been recommended in doses of two tablets. After several years, "extra strength" tablets were made available, although the suggested dosage was still two tablets. Then we could have 500 mg per tablet instead of 325 mg. All the years we were being advised to take 650 mg, we really could have been taking 1,000 mg. Most people in our society will never take more medication than is recommended. How many people had severe pain during the 650 mg years that 1,000 mg would have helped or stopped?

Knowing that the public has spent many years in the past with inadequate dosage, we must ask these questions: How much pain reliever can we really take? During the many years that these products have been on the market, why couldn't adults have had a weight-to-dosage table like that put on the same medication for children? These questions are at the root of our need to take control of our own migraine destiny. We have effectively been denied the right to use our common sense. No wonder we don't know how to handle these headaches. We don't even know how much pain reliever we can really take.

To get a handle on this problem, let's look at the amount of acetaminophen that the drug companies claim is "safe and effective" and devise a weight-to-dosage table. The de facto basic claim is that two tablets are an adult dose, even if they are extra strength. That would translate to 1,000 mg for any adult. If we were to devise a table, we would need a minimum adult weight to establish as a base line for a calculation. Even though there are millions of healthy adults who weigh substantially less than 100 lbs, this weight is close to the adult minimum. It is an easy number to divide into the 1,000 mg dose that the pharmaceutical companies now claim any adult can take. For those of us who weigh more than 100 lbs, these numbers give a nice 1 lb to 10 mg ratio as the basis for our table.

We also need to design a comparable formula to use for ibuprofen. The tablets contain 200 mg, and the recommended dose is, again, two tablets. This would be 400 mg for our basic 100 lb person. In determining an amount that is effective on migraines, it appears that a 1 lb to 5 mg ratio is effective. That is 500 mg for a 100 lb individual, or three tablets (which is a little stronger than the base line formula at 600 mg, but you would have to cut a tablet in half to arrive at 500 mg for a 100-pounder). These are easy numbers to figure in your head, and they work out well at higher weights.

Let's take a moment to see which pain reliever you should use and how much you should take.

IBUPROFEN: With the early-stage symptoms described previously, ibuprofen is the medication of choice. The ibuprofen formula is 5 mg per lb of body weight. If you weigh 120 lbs, for example, you will need 600 mg, or three tablets at 200 mg each. Ibuprofen pain relievers include Advil, Datril, Motrin, Nuprin, and generic brands; all work equally well. At the early-cure stage we are still attempting to trick the system, so take this with a little orange juice. The reason for using ibuprofen for the early headache is that it works very well on normal headaches and early migraines but acetaminophen works best on the full migraine. You need to save your Tylenol exposure in case you are not successful at the early stage and need it later for the full migraine.

ACETAMINOPHEN: This is the most effective medication for the most advanced stage—the fully developed migraine. Nothing reaches down into the depths of the stomach to open the passage to the small intestine like acetaminophen. The formula is 10 mg per lb of body weight. If you weigh 120 lbs, for example, you will need 1,200 mg.

Fortunately, acetaminophen comes in both 325 mg and 500 mg tablets, so you can buy the size that comes closest to a multiple of your weight. Brand names include Tylenol and Anacin III, and generic non-aspirin pain relievers; all are identically effective. Take with orange juice. I have recommended that you not use acetaminophen at this stage. But when you become experienced at curing your migraine at this level and are confident you won't need to follow up with more pain reliever, it's certainly okay to use acetaminophen for the early cure.

IBUPROFEN-ACETAMINOPHEN COMBINATION: To avoid taking a large amount of either pain reliever, you or your doctor may feel it is best to combine for the strong dosage required to unlock the passage to the small intestine. If you use a combination of pain relievers, simply apply one-half of your weight to the formula for ibuprofen and one-half of your weight to the formula for acetaminophen. Take with orange juice. I recommend combining pain relievers when both types have been used within the last 12 hours.

ALTERNATE PAIN RELIEVERS: You may develop a habit of taking one pain reliever more often than the other. Try to balance your usage to lessen the exposure to either medication. One of my little lessons in life (and I learned 'em all the hard way) is that anything, even water and air, will develop complications if used excessively.

Regardless of whether you feel that you are eliminating an early migraine or just a normal headache, the pain reliever should be taken with a small amount of orange juice (¼ cup). After the analgesic has had 10 or 15 minutes to enter the bloodstream and you *definitely* feel that the headache is over, drink a full glass of juice. This will continue to trick the stomach out of secreting its own gastric acid and will offset a possible relapse.

With the lesser headache you are still attempting to trick your stomach out of acid secretion with a mildly acidic drink. These instructions will change dramatically with the full-stage migraine. Then you will use only enough liquid to swallow the pain reliever. The chapter titled The Full Migraine Dry Stomach Sponge Cure explains the need to keep the volume of liquid as low as possible.

Now you have seen how an early-stage migraine (or normal headache) is relieved by common analgesics. It's no big surprise that these two products will relieve a normal headache. But it may be new information that a migraine can often be avoided by normal measures if it's caught early. It may also be news that opening the stomach plays a significant role. The part that a pain reliever plays in emptying the stomach at the early stage becomes crucial in relieving the total migraine. The important things to know are how to recognize the headache as early as possible, and how much pain reliever is right for you.

DISCLAIMER

At this point, I would like to remind you that I am not a doctor. *Master Your Migraine* has been compiled entirely from my personal experiences, insights, and conclusions, and it is only intended as a guideline for fellow sufferers. The purpose of this manual is solely to help other victims begin a learning process to control their own migraines. In doing so, I may have recommended larger doses, depending on your weight, than are stated on pain reliever containers. I would therefore also recommend that each of you discuss these dosages, and all other portions of this manual, with your professional health care specialist.

IX

Stomach Physiology and The Dry Stomach Sponge

After many years of migraine nausea, I developed the notion that the headache was caused by stomach acid instead of the reverse. Concentrating on that thesis, finding a possible cure meant focusing on ways to alter the stomach's natural tendency to fill with acid. Every possible way of handling the acid was tried, including neutralization, prescription acid duct antihistamines, and voluntary regurgitation. All met with limited success. The next idea was to somehow assist the acid to continue on its way down through the system. This worked! By opening the sphincter to the small intestine, I could move the poison from the stomach into the lower digestive tract.

Some questions may come immediately to mind. Why is it necessary to squeegee out the stomach? And why doesn't the stomach simply empty completely after it has been opened into the small intestine? The answer in both cases is the evolved design for digestion, which traps foods that are not fully broken down. This design also traps *us* into these very severe headaches.

There are contributing factors within the stomach that help to lock the system into a migraine. Our stomachs have the ability to select different food items for digestion. We have all had indigestion, where something eaten several hours earlier is still being experienced later in the day (like the taste of pepperoni, celery, or lettuce), but other items eaten at the same meal may no longer be noticed. It seems as though little hands are at work picking and choosing what must leave and what must stay for more processing. We could attribute this strange

38

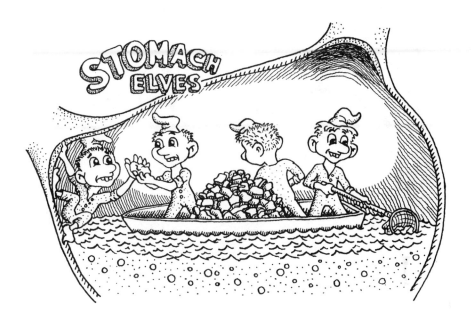

phenomenon to the Stomach Elves, but they will eventually have to join Santa and the Tooth Fairy in mythdom.

Two characteristics of digestion share the honor of being both the blessings that allow all foods to be processed together, regardless of consistency, and the menaces that trigger the migraine.

The first is the *shape of the stomach*, especially the lower portion. When the stomach is viewed from the front, it appears to be lying on its side. The connection to the remainder of the digestive tract is higher than the bottom extent. In other words, there is a sag or holding area lower than the exit from the stomach. This makes it possible to leave the harder-to-digest foods behind and pass the easier ones on to the next stage of processing in the small intestine.

The second mechanism is *specific gravity*. Simply put, all substances have a different weight if compared at the same volume. We have all seen the commercial for liquid drain cleaner. The cleaner is poured into a sink full of water to unclog the drain. The television viewer may wonder why it goes to the bottom instead of dispersing in the water. And how does it displace the water that is far down in the drain? The answer to both questions is specific gravity. Although the drain cleaner is a liquid like the water, it is an acid and has a higher specific gravity. In other words, it is simply heavier and can push aside the water in the drainpipe, find its way to the clog, and dissolve it.

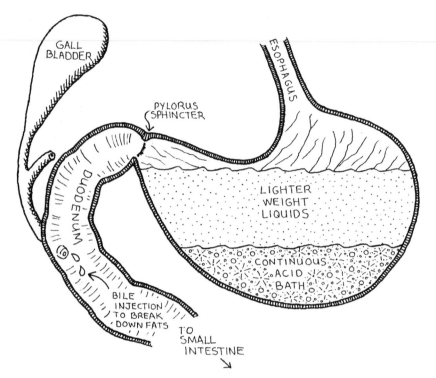

VARYING PHYSICAL CHARACTERISTICS CAN CAUSE BILE INTRODUCTION TO THE STOMACH

Stomach acid is also heavier than water and works in much the same way as drain cleaner. It goes to the lowest possible location and breaks down or dissolves whatever it comes in contact with. This works well in a stomach designed with a holding area lower than the exit opening. The miracle of the design is that it can hold certain foods in a prolonged acid bath until they are ready to be accepted by the small intestine. Nature spent eons perfecting this shape. It is one of the basics for life in higher organisms. Unfortunately, this beautiful creation of nature turns into an equally menacing one when coping with a headache.

When the stomach has initiated a CAP episode, it is then trapped within that event. The acid cannot escape, and even when neutralized, enough poisoning chemical components are still present to keep the cycle intact. The acid stays in the stomach holding area and can only be removed by the "dry sponge" method.

The term *dry sponge* has a double meaning. First, it means to sponge the stomach dry by soaking up the acid with a substance that will use the acid in a positive way. The sponge removes the acid as the acid breaks down the sponging material. After the sponging medium is broken down, it then becomes a source of badly needed nutrition for the blood system. It replaces the poison that has been the only thing available to the bloodstream due to the CAP lock. Second, the term means that the sponging substance must be eaten dry (without drinking anything). Naturally, if you're trying to soak up the liquid that is already present, you should not drink anything. Any new liquid will only float on top of the acid and complicate the soaking process. The sponging substance will be suspended in the lighter weight liquid, and the acid/poison will remain intact and continue to maintain the migraine lock. If you drink anything with the sponging food, the cure will not work.

An important point to remember is that the opening to the small intestine is on the right side of the stomach. When working the cure, it will help the stomach to empty if you lie on your right side. It is not critical to do this—the cure will work anyway—but it's a good thing to know when your cure needs a little assistance.

X

The Full Migraine Dry Stomach Sponge Cure

Before you start the full cure, you must have made the decision that your headache has gone beyond the point of normal treatment discussed in the early-cure section. This decision is not very difficult. At a certain degree of misery, you will simply assess yourself and make the determination that the stomach sponge is now necessary.

To help in making that decision, consider whether you have progressed to the point of having the following symptoms to at least a moderate degree: pain in your temples and eyes, tension in the back of your head and neck, head pain, and nausea. If all of these exist, you have become a candidate for the dry sponge.

You needn't be concerned about making this decision. It won't hurt to use the full cure, even if a lesser measure would work. On the other hand, your headache cannot be too severe for the sponge to work. After you have had some experience with working the sponge, you will develop an instinct for that point of agony which requires its use. You may think you are in such a state of misery that nothing can help. My personal experience with hundreds of migraines has shown that the worse the headache becomes, the better the dry sponge works, and no migraine is too bad.

The cure for a full-scale migraine starts with the early-migraine cure, but with two changes. The first difference is to use acetaminophen instead of ibuprofen, because acetaminophen is considerably more effective. The second difference is to drink only enough liquid to swallow the pain reliever. When the full cure has become necessary, you are beyond the point that drinking a mildly acidic liquid will be helpful. Now that it is time to sponge your stomach, the extra liquid simply requires more sponging.

1. *Neutralize or eliminate the acid.* You have decided that you are sick beyond a normal headache, with nausea to some degree, and it's time to work the full cure. Now you must analyze how much acid is in your stomach by how nauseated you are. This will determine the next course of action.

On a nausea scale of one to ten (with ten being an immediate run to the bathroom to throw up), if you are anything higher than a five, the cure will be greatly assisted if your stomach is emptied. I characterize the nausea level of five as the beginning of the feeling that throwing up is becoming inevitable. If you have passed the point of no return with nausea, either wait to throw up, tickle your tonsils, or use whatever means are at your disposal to encourage it to happen.

This is where you must live up to your responsibility to yourself as a migraine sufferer. You must take a proactive approach toward the inevitable and shorten the duration of your agony. Usually a quick look at the tray under your refrigerator will handle the situation. If that doesn't work, come look at mine.

All jokes aside, when you are a migraine sufferer, purging your stomach is a fact of life. The idea of doing it voluntarily may be foreign to you, so I will give you a couple of pointers. First, this is no time to be weak willed. When it's time to let it rip, don't hold back—bring it up from your toes. You want to clean your stomach out as well as it can be done. So keep at it until nothing more comes up, and then heave once more "for the Gipper."

Emptying the stomach is the best way to start the cure. It removes a large portion of the problem, requiring less antacid and less sponging, but it will not cure the headache by itself. After the stomach is empty and the acid is gone, there will be some relief for a short period. Do not be fooled by this false sense of relief; the acid and the headache will return. The dry sponge will still work, even if the stomach is not empty, but it will require more sponging.

Now that you have either thrown up or have decided that you are not sick enough to need to, you are are ready to proceed with the cure by neutralizing your acidity. By the time the more advanced migraine has developed, even if you have thrown up you will still have some acid to neutralize.

When neutralizing your acid for the early cure (the normal headache), you learned to simply take the recommended dosage listed on the antacid container. When working the full cure, if you have emptied your stomach the recommended dosage will still be adequate. On the other hand, I take a dose and a half if I am working the full cure without an empty stomach.

After taking the antacid, you must wait three minutes for neutralization to occur. Sometimes taking an antacid will cause vomiting if you are nauseous. This little wait is to allow enough time to see if that happens. If you do vomit within the three minutes, simply take it again. If you throw up the antacid a second time, forget it.

Keep in mind that taking an antacid can be overdone, and it does not play as important a part in the cure as the pain reliever or the dry sponge. If you do not have access to an antacid, the sponge will work without it but may require more sponging food and a little more time.

While the acid level is lowered and any still remaining has been neutralized, it's time to unlock the stomach.

2. *Unlock the stomach.* Take the pain reliever to relax the cramp and unlock the stomach passage to the small intestine. As mentioned earlier, keep the volume of liquid as low as possible by drinking only enough to swallow the pain reliever.

• *Acetaminophen.* The dosage is the same as the early cure, 10 mg per 1 lb of body weight. You can easily figure your own dosage. Simply add a zero to your weight and divide that number by the milligrams in the tablets. After taking the acetaminophen with a small amount of liquid (¼ cup), wait five minutes for it to begin to be absorbed. Waiting gives the pain reliever a head start toward the bloodstream. Otherwise, some of the analgesic may be sponged up during the next step and not given a chance to do its work.

The pain reliever will act on the nervous system and open the lock at the base of the stomach. Do not expect the pain to vanish simply by taking the acetaminophen. As we all know, OTC pain relievers will not stop a migraine.

• *Ibuprofen.* Although the second choice, it will work effectively to open the stomach for those who cannot use acetaminophen. Take the same dosage as recommended in the early cure (5 mg per lb of body weight). Figure your own dosage by multiplying your weight by 5 and dividing the total by 200 (OTC ibuprofen comes only in 200 mg tablets).

• *Acetaminophen-ibuprofen combination.* If you need an extra strong dose, it may be best to combine the pain relievers. Do not resort to higher doses until you see whether the recommended dose works. Then refer to the Final Attempt chapter to proceed further.

DO NOT REPEAT DOSAGES: At this point, something must be said about large amounts of acetaminophen. High doses can cause liver malfunction, and death has resulted on rare occasions. However, it takes about thirty regular tablets in the bloodstream in a single day for the average person to exceed the danger point.

On the other hand, you stand a better chance of taking a dangerous amount of pain reliever by strict adherence to recommended doses. You can follow the labeled dose into the trap of overdosing. If you take the recommended amount every few hours and don't end your headache, you can grossly overdose in a 24-hour period. In my opinion, it is a better option to take the somewhat stronger weight-table dose one time and end your migraine. Once again, I am not a doctor, and I urge you to discuss this opinion with your physician.

3. *Use the dry stomach sponge.* This is the best trick I have found after a decade of trying gastric acid duct antihistamines, alkaloids, coating agents, added acids, stomach purges, and of course everything suggested by all the doctors.

There are several high-carbohydrate foods that will sponge out your stomach and resupply nutrition to your bloodstream, thus ending your migraine. All of them but one can be found at any grocery or convenience store. The one you cannot find at a store is a special muffin mix that I have formulated for myself and call the Migraine Muffin. It is designed with natural tricking, absorbing, and digestion-enhancing properties to specifically target your migraine. An order form is included in this manual if you would like to order the mix and make the muffins fresh at home.

There may be many foods that will work other than those discussed here. These work very well, so I have not experimented with a lot of other absorbing agents. This is where I need help from my readers. I have found the basic answer to the migraine lock, but we all still need help from each other to continue to discover new variations on my migraine-elimination system.

Any new dry sponge foods must provide easily converted complex carbohydrate (starch) to replace the poison in the blood. They must also be edible without liquid and still have room to absorb more fluid. Foods such as rice, pasta, and mashed potatoes have absorbed all the moisture they can hold, and therefore they do not sponge efficiently. Conversely, puffed grains such as puffed wheat, rice cakes, and popcorn float like styrofoam atop the moisture and will not absorb it. The following sponging materials are the old standbys that I normally use. These are tried and true dry sponge foods.

• *Bread.* Have available a hearty, heavy-grained bread such as 100 percent stone ground whole wheat and bran. (A couple of favorite

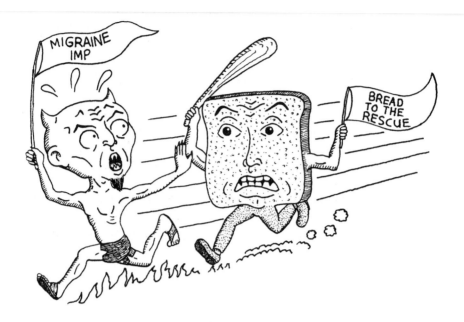

brands are Grants Farm and Oroweat.) Most breads are very good at sponging, although I have never tried white bread. It may not have enough fiber to offset constipation caused by the large amounts necessary to sponge the stomach. When choosing a bread, look for bran or whole grain, and avoid bread with nuts, sunflower seeds, wheat berries, or anything else hard in the bread. Dense substances cause more acid to be introduced to break them down, which defeats the bread's sponging ability.

Eat four to six slices dry, depending on your weight and how full your stomach is. Do not drink any liquid with the bread. This is the hard part. It is difficult to swallow anything when you are nauseous, but each slice goes down more easily than the one before.

To make this task more palatable, put the bread in the microwave for about ten seconds to warm and moisten it before eating. I have been asked if toasted bread will work as well. The answer is yes, but toasting won't help. Since you cannot put anything on the toast, it will be harder to eat than regular bread.

The bread will soak up the poison and carry it down the digestive tract into the small intestine. The migraine is usually gone by the end of the last slice, so don't give up early. You may think that nothing is happening during the first four slices, and you may want to abort the task. For me, at 160 lbs, the headache lets go during the last half of the fifth slice. The migraine releases very suddenly, so hang in there and keep munching at the bread.

An interesting thing happens immediately after the migraine lifts. You feel euphoric, almost giddy or high. This may indicate that the migraine pain has produced endorphens that linger for some time after the headache has been eliminated.

The transition can take place within as little as five minutes, but it usually takes between ten and fifteen. In this short period you will have gone from extreme misery to a light-headed sense of well-being so rapidly that I describe it as "reality whiplash."

My personal best time for a start-to-finish cure for a full migraine is seventeen minutes. The average cure takes thirty-five to forty minutes. As you can see, playing with migraines has been a favorite pastime.

Persons weighing under 120 lbs may need only four slices. Larger persons, over 170 lbs, may need to eat a sixth slice. A rule of thumb is one slice per 30 lbs of body weight. Use wide-loaf bread to get the correct volume.

• *Potatoes.* Their starch absorbs stomach acid and provides fresh complex carbohydrates for the blood just as bread does. You can cook them any way you like as long as you eat three or four large potatoes (4 in × 2 in), depending on your weight and how much acid is in your stomach when you start. Like the bread, potatoes must be eaten dry. Do not put anything on them for flavor except a small amount of salt. Any toppings will pollute the dry sponge, but you are not very concerned with taste when you are in the grip of a migraine anyway.

There are several quick and easy ways to prepare the potatoes. The easiest method is to toss them into a microwave and then eat the soft pulp with a spoon. Regardless of the method you choose, *do not eat the skins;* they require additional stomach acid to digest.

My favorite potato cure is french fries. Although they are cooked in oil, they still work great. They should be made from fresh potatoes. It has been my experience that frozen fries do not work as well. My guess is that freezing breaks down the cell structure and alters their absorbency.

The fries cannot be soggy. They must be cooked in very hot oil to lower the oil saturation. Use a deep fryer, such as the Fry Daddy brand, that is designed specifically for cooking fries. This ensures that they are cooked at the proper temperature (360–400°F), sealing the fry and lowering oil absorption.

Fries should be prepared in a high-quality oil that is low in saturated fat. Absolutely no animal fat (lard) can be used or the fries become a trigger. A high-quality oil is important for other reasons. It assists the carbohydrate in providing some quick nutrition for replacement of the poison in the blood. There may also be some value in coating the stomach with the oil.

Choose your cooking oil carefully by reading and comparing labels. The percentages of saturated fat and cholesterol are listed on the label. The lower the numbers, the better. At the time of the latest rewrite of this manual, Canola oil had the best health statistics and has worked well for me.

Potatoes cooked by other methods should work as well, as long as nothing is added and no animal fat is used.

• *Crackers*. This is Melissa's Cure. Melissa is my daughter, and she had her first full-scale migraine when spending the summer at my house at the age of 10. (She would insist that she was 10½.)

One morning we were preoccupied and forgot to eat breakfast. Melissa soon developed a full-scale migraine. She threw up every sponging substance we tried, as well as the antacid and acetaminophen. I was at a loss. I had never tried this cure on a child. I didn't know if she had expelled all of the pain reliever, so I was reluctant to give her more. She had vomited six times in five hours, and I had tried a new trick each time. Now I was all out of tricks.

Melissa had been with me all summer while I was working on the migraine manual. She discusses things on a very mature level and had been involved in the book with me, and now Daddy couldn't cure her. There is no more helpless feeling than watching your child suffer, but this was even worse. I was about to lose face with my daughter, who at this age still thought I was Superman.

Then we thought of it at the same time: "Crackers!" We said it simultaneously. She started eating them and, thank God, they stayed down. She was better almost instantly—*much* better, almost well. I had not felt it was safe to allow her to take more pain reliever. She was content to feel improvement as she leisurely crunched crackers for a couple more hours. When enough time had passed, she did it right and took the Tylenol, followed by more crackers. At this point she took no more antacid, because I didn't want to risk making her throw up again. She went through a sleeve and a half of crackers that day, but she got well, totally well, in the course of an afternoon. Best of all, I still got to be Superman for another year, or maybe two!

The moral of this story is: If you can't keep any sponging food down, try Melissa's Cure. If you keep some crackers around for this purpose, I would recommend the new no-fat ones, and it would be good to go with no-salt too, if they are ever in the same cracker.

48

• *Migraine Muffins.* Mentioned earlier, these are specially formulated bran muffins designed for enhanced absorption. They also contain acid-tricking properties and ingredients that speed digestion.

In my experience the muffins probably work best, in addition to being tastier, although the advantage of the muffins is theoretical and not yet proven. The bread works quite well if you do not have difficulty eating it dry. Bread is easy to obtain and works well enough that some sufferers may have success with little or no pain reliever.

Save the potatoes as a backup in the event that you're having trouble getting rid of an especially difficult migraine (addressed in Final Attempt). Potatoes are a safe starchy meal to eat for that completely well feeling, after your headache leaves and you begin to feel better. If you wait until the headache has lifted before eating your fries, you can have all the ketchup on them that your lil ol' heart desires. Now, that's some incentive, huh?

While eating the last two slices of bread, pay close attention to how you feel. A hunger pang or gurgling sensation in your digestive tract (usually contractions emptying your stomach) will indicate that your stomach has opened and food is going into the small intestine. You will learn to anticipate and appreciate that feeling. Surprisingly, after eating all that food, you will be hungry very soon after finishing the last of the bread or fries. When you feel the hunger pangs, you are rapidly becoming well and it is time for the next step.

4. *Replenish your system with non-triggering food and drink.* When you feel better, it is time for that huge plate of fries with ketchup. You're really going to want to drink something now. If you're sure that the headache is completely gone, then have a little orange juice with your fries, and enjoy them. *You deserve it—you have just mastered your migraine!*

5. *Stimulate the system with caffeine when the head pain is gone.* Caffeine can often help accomplish that fully recovered feeling after the head pain is completely gone. A little system pick-me-up will help to speed up the digestion process and move poisons out of the body. As it takes effect, you may have some diarrhea within a few hours after curing your headache. This is a result of expelling the acid poison in your lower digestive tract. Caffeine helps clean out your system faster.

Remember that having caffeine during a migraine will not assist in ridding it, as it sometimes does a lesser headache. A stimulant will worsen a migraine by increasing the power of the cranial cramp. This is a problem with pain relievers, such as Anacin and Excedrin, that contain caffeine as a main ingredient.

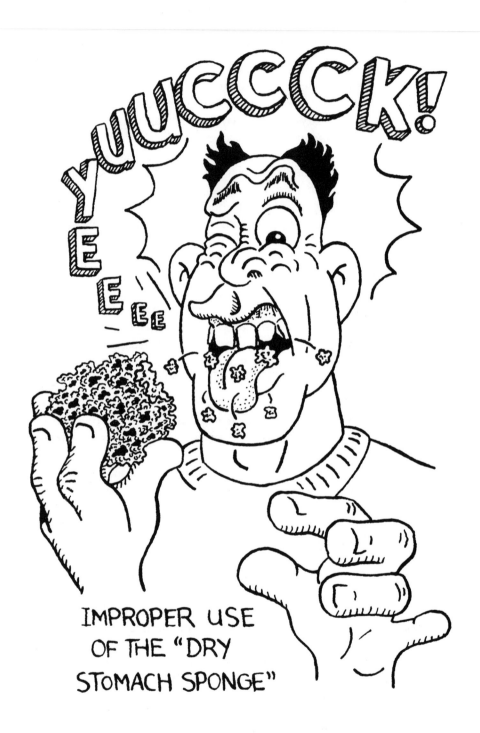

Caffeine is only beneficial in the following instances:

• When you normally have caffeine daily, have not had your regular amount for the day, and are ridding yourself of a normal headache or early-stage migraine;

• When a full-stage migraine has been dry sponged and is completely gone;

• When the migraine has been dry sponged and you are much improved, but there is a little headache remaining and you have not had your normal daily amount of caffeine due to your migraine. The lingering need for the caffeine can continue to cause a withdrawal headache.

6. *Take a hot shower or bath*. Let the water soak your head, neck, shoulers and back. Then get a good massage. There is no describing how good it feels on those cramp-weary muscles. You may want to keep a good masseuse on retainer.

When you have a migraine, are working the cure, or are just relaxing after the cure has worked, remember that the stomach opening to the small intestine is on your right side, and gravity will help empty the stomach contents into the small intestine if you lie on your right side.

Unfortunately, even when you are well you are not out of danger of recurrence, because you may be in a migraine-prone phase or cycle. Migraines can return easily, so proceed carefully after achieving that wonderful feeling of relief. Never take being well for granted. Migraine relief is continuously earned. A potential migraine always lurks within the next snack, meal, or tense moment. Learn all of the tricks and triggers, and remember them at all times. It is especially important to keep them in mind when purchasing your groceries. This is one of my little rules: If it is not in the house, it's a lot harder to eat. Always be cautious about what you eat, especially those late-night snacks while watching the tube. They are the main cause of the dreaded migraine during sleep, discussed in a later chapter.

A QUICK REVIEW OF THE CURE

1. Deplete the stomach acid.
   • Throw up if moderately nauseous
   • Neutralize your acidity; wait three minutes
2. Unlock the stomach.
   • Take your weight-table dosage of acetaminophen (10 mg × body weight) or other pain reliever; wait five minutes
3. Work the dry stomach sponge.
   • Eat 6 to 8 oz carbohydrate (4 to 6 slices of bread at 1 slice per 30 lbs); eat dry (no liquid); the headache will subside quickly as

you finish.

4. Replenish the remaining weak feeling by replacing the poison in the bloodstream with non-triggering food and drink.
5. Have caffeine to stimulate your system after the head pain leaves.
6. Soak sore muscles in a hot shower or bath, and get a massage if possible.

HIATAL HERNIA WARNING

A hiatal hernia is an abnormality in the structure of the stomach area. If the hernia is in a critical position, in or near the esophagus, it can cause difficulty in swallowing. This problem can lead to choking or vomiting. If you have ever been diagnosed with a hiatal hernia by a medical practitioner, or if you suspect that you may have one, do not try this cure without consulting your health care professional.

If you have ever had a problem with choking while eating, or have had a need to drink large amounts of liquid to assist swallowing, do not try this cure dry. You need to have medical attention for your problem. If your doctor tells you that your condition will not allow eating without liquid, do not attempt to use the dry stomach sponge.

With the permission of your health care specialist, you can try an altered, less-efficient version of the cure. You can try acid duct antihistamines to help stop acid flow, then dilute the poison already in your stomach with tricking drink and sponging food. Drink large amounts of orange juice, or another mildly acidic drink, to assist in swallowing the bread, potatoes, or other sponging food. Larger amounts and more time will be needed to clear the stomach. It will not actually be sponged, but if you have managed to open your stomach with the pain reliever, the acidic poison will be diluted and eventually carried away.

XI

Final Attempt

Y ou have followed the process previously outlined, but the cure has
still not worked. A few more measures are necessary.

Make sure you have allowed enough time for the dry sponge to
work. If the pain is not decreasing as you finish the last slice of bread
for your weight, try a couple more slices. This is a lot of bread, but it is
not harmful in any way, and it's certainly better than having a migraine.
If you still have a headache after you have eaten a few more slices of
bread, you must take additional steps.

Apparently you started the cure with a large amount of acid that
will need more sponging. This is a good time to continue the dry
sponge cure using potatoes. Pull out all the stops and continue with
a large plate of fries made from three or four potatoes. At this point
you still need to eat the sponge food dry. Sorry, no ketchup.

If the pain and nausea persist, the only thing left to try is an increase
of pain reliever. Discuss this part with your professional health care
specialist. This manual is written from a personal perspective, and a
practice that has apparently been safe and beneficial for one person
may not be so for everyone.

With the approval of medical counsel, increasing the pain reliever
is more safely done if a different product is used than the one taken
earlier. The point of using another type is to lessen the amount of any
one chemical in the body. An overdose of pain reliever is more serious
than the headache, even though there is a profound sense of despera-
tion during the pain. If you have used acetaminophen, now it is time

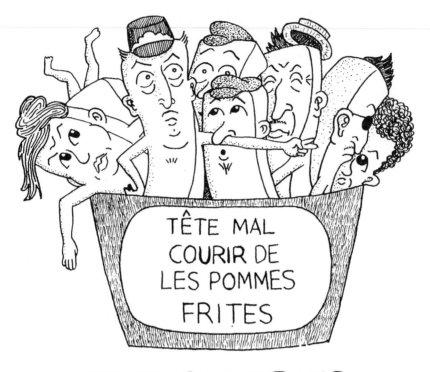

TÊTE MAL
COURIR DE
LES POMMES
FRITES

FRENCH FRIES

to use ibuprofen. Never use aspirin. It is inferior to all other products and thins the blood too much when used in large amounts.

Use only one regular tablet as a boost to open the stomach passage. Wait 10 to 20 minutes to notice the effect. When adding extra pain reliever, never exceed half of the original amount recommended earlier in the full-cure portion of the manual. For example, the recommended dosage for ibuprofen discussed earlier is 5 mg for every pound of body weight, e.g., 800 mg for a 160-lb person. One-half of that amount would be 400 mg for a 160-lb person.

If you see that you always need to resort to an increase of pain reliever to finally eliminate your migraine, you are probably not taking enough at the beginning to open your stomach. Try to find the minimum amount of extra pain reliever that will open your stomach to the small intestine, allowing the stomach to be sponged. Once you have found how much it takes to get that result, add that amount to the other pain reliever at the beginning of the cure, when it will be more effective. It will work even better than when you use it in the final attempt, and you may not need quite as much. You will not have added any sponging food at that point to dilute the potency of the analgesic.

If you still have a headache after eating extra bread and/or potatoes and after taking extra pain reliever, you may have something else to consider. In this case it is time to go to a medical professional and have tests run on other possible neurological problems. If this layman's home cure has not worked, I heartily recommend that you seek professional medical attention.

When discussing your problem with a medical professional, you may want to ask for help in controlling your acid secretion. Acid duct antihistamines that will dry up the acid flow and assist the stomach sponge can be purchased OTC or prescribed by your doctor. The prescription drugs are sold under the brand names of Zantac and Tagamet. Zantac is newer and is usually the more effective of the two. Less potent versions of acid duct antihistamines are now available OTC, under the brand names Zantac, Pepcid, and Tagamet II. In my personal experience, I have found that these antihistamines work; I have used them all in the developmental stages of my cure. Get as much advice as possible from your doctor, and if you have any reservations about what you're being told, get more than one opinion. Always remember that doctors are just people too.

XII

Curing the Migraine Before It Starts

Y ou have seen how to treat the early symptoms and the full-stage migraine by getting to know the headache and directly addressing the cause. Now you can take this knowledge a step further and stop the headache in advance.

At times a headache is unavoidable even though you know what causes it. Often when you are a guest at someone's home, at a formal function, or at an outing with friends, you are unable to control the menu. In these cases it is important to have a working grasp of the tricks and triggers as well as all variations of the cure.

One variation of the cure is to use it in advance of the headache. For example, at a dinner party hosted by your boss, you see that the main course is roast beef, with milk as the only drink. You are fully aware that this is a migraine waiting to happen. You are in the difficult position of displeasing your boss or instigating a severe headache. Many sufferers regularly find themselves in this kind of situation, with no other options available, and submit to the pressure and to the migraine.

There is another course of action. Open the stomach sphincter, either before the meal or immediately after it, so that the stomach does not bottle up and start the cyclical acid flow. Simply take the pain reliever before eating the meal or soon after you have finished it. The pain reliever will keep the stomach open to the digestive tract and inhibit the tendency to trap the acid and start the CAP effect.

A word of caution: Do not take this principle to its extreme. Do not assume that if some works, more will work better. By following

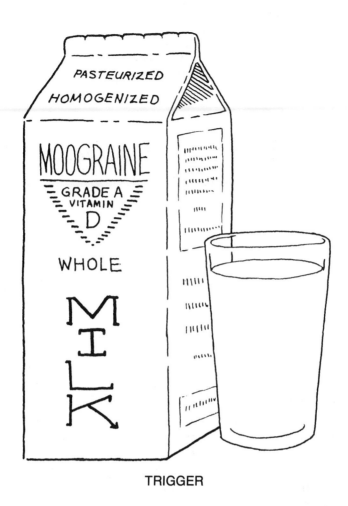

TRIGGER

that logic, a desperate sufferer might take pain reliever before every meal. This can cause serious side effects, as you give your body too much of one chemical. This can also create a tolerance to the analgesic, which will diminish its potency for future effectiveness. Cure your headache in advance only when there is no other avenue of escape. As before, "Moderation in everything . . ."—you know the rest.

XIII

The Migraine During Sleep

A major problem for the migraine sufferer is the migraine that develops during sleep. As the head pain builds, your sleep becomes
more and more restless until you awaken with a full-scale migraine.
Obviously, the early stage has passed without giving you a chance to
recognize it and has not allowed you the opportunity to take some
corrective action. This is one of the more pressing difficulties in controlling migraines. Luckily, in light of what you have now learned
from this manual, you can approach this problem from a few different directions.

First, understanding all areas of the migraine is the solution. In this
instance, be aware of consuming trigger foods before bedtime. The
main culprit is the late-night snack. There is nothing worse than eating
trigger foods, especially fatty ones like ice cream, pizza, or meat, before
going to bed. Watch closely what you eat in the evening hours, then
wait at least one hour after the last food has been consumed before
retiring. This allows you enough time to see if any early symptoms
will develop.

During the wait between the last food and bedtime, pay very close
attention to any early warnings. If you notice even the slightest sign,
do not hesitate to act immediately. Work the early cure, using either
acetaminophen or ibuprofen. Take acetaminophen if you are sure you
have eaten or drunk a positive trigger. Using the more reliable pain
reliever is important when you have only one chance to stop the headache before you are asleep and it's too late. You can use ibuprofen if

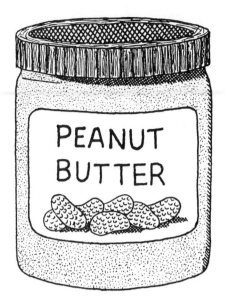

TRIGGER

you feel you are having only mild early symptoms.

It is critical that you not let denial cloud your better judgment. Many people who suffer from headaches think that a slight headache will simply go away if they go to sleep. Although this may work on the everyday headache, a migraine almost always becomes worse as you sleep.

After you have learned your triggers, you will know when one has been eaten. Or you may have a history of a particular food being a sure-bet culprit. When you are sure that you have consumed a trigger, curing the headache in advance is an appropriate action.

Once again orange juice is a good bedtime drink. It is something good to have with any late-night snack or by itself, whether or not any pain is present. If you are working the early cure or the cure in advance and have taken a pain reliever with a small amount (2 oz) of orange juice, wait twenty minutes. If your symptoms do not develop further and you feel the original pain subside, drink a full glass of orange juice. If you have eaten a trigger but do not feel that you need a pain reliever, it is still a good idea to have a glass of orange juice before bed. Other non-sweet, mildly acidic drinks can be substituted. Just consider them bedtime migraine insurance.

There are a couple of other possible triggers that deserve a quick look. One is sleeping in a room that is too warm. This is easy to fix (if you can get your significant other to cooperate). Always set your thermostat at 65° before bedtime.

The other culprit is dreaming intensely. Sometimes a dream that is nightmarish may set the migraine machinery in motion. This is one of those chicken or egg dilemmas. You don't really know if it's the food you ate at supper that is causing the migraine or if the rich, spicy, or gas-producing foods have started an intense dream. If this is not actually started by a trigger food and is caused by the dream, it is probably just your average tension migraine. The body responds to stress caused by a bad dream just as it does to that brought on by any of life's problems while awake.

Unfortunately, there is no easy way out of this. It is difficult to control dreams. The only dream-altering tactic may be to avoid things which you have found to cause them, such as troublesome foods and stress in your life.

Regardless of what caused your headache to escalate while you were asleep, when you awaken with your migraine in full force, go into immediate action and start the full cure. The sooner you get out of bed and cure your headache, the more sleep you will get that night. Going back to sleep and hoping it will go away is not an option.

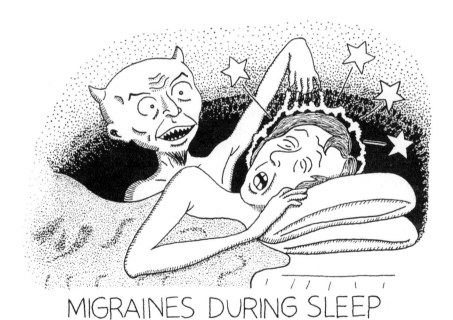

MIGRAINES DURING SLEEP

XIV

The Migraine Triggered by Lack of Sleep

Another sleep-related problem with this painful malady is the migraine caused by sleep deprivation. Occasionally you may need to spend long hours awake due to your job, long drives, sick children or any of life's many requirements. We all must pass up our beauty sleep at times, but the outcome may be significantly different for migraine victims. The lack of sleep can not only cause a headache, it can create another vicious cycle, which compounds the cleanup process of the home cure.

After being awake for 16 to 20 hours, you may experience an entirely new migraine symptom. The first indication is the frequent need to urinate, with only 10- to 20-minute intervals between trips to the bathroom. This will happen even though you have not consumed any liquid. Your body has gone into shock from sleep deprivation and is rapidly eliminating water from its system. In other words, you are dehydrating.

Within minutes of the start of water elimination, usually after the second or third immediate trip to the bathroom, the sphincter at the base of the stomach cramps and locks the acids in the stomach. The CAP process has begun, and the more familiar symptoms will soon follow. The muscles begin to cramp around the upper spine, through the back of the neck, and around the skull. The migraine starts instantly. The onset of this migraine is the second fastest that you can have, beaten only by the one started by hunger.

Now that the headache process has been set up and you are again

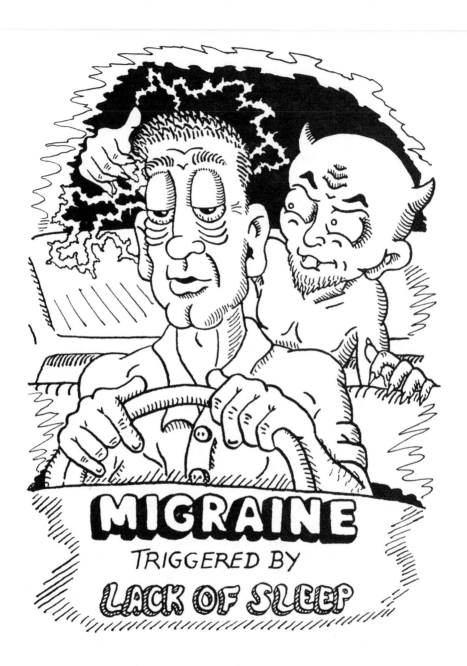

MIGRAINE

TRIGGERED BY

LACK OF SLEEP

in the abyss of pain, it becomes apparent that more than the migraine must be dealt with. A catch in the cure has become evident: sleep deprivation is causing the headache, and you cannot sleep because of the pain.

THE SOLUTION: There is a way out of this dilemma, but it is a bit complex. The sufferer must understand it well in advance of the headache. This is true of all migraines, but especially so with the one caused by sleep deprivation. You must not only know the dry stomach sponge well enough to work it blindfolded by pain, you must also be armed with the extra particulars involved with this lack-of-sleep dilemma.

As soon as the rapid liquid elimination starts, the headache must be addressed immediately. In this instance, it is your very first early warning symptom. If a pain reliever is taken after the second or third rapid urination, before any pain has begun, the entire headache process can be averted. The stomach will remain open to the small intestine after the sphincter cramp is relaxed by the analgesic. The cyclical acid flow will not be allowed to bottle, and the pain will be stopped before it has a chance to start.

Sometimes early warnings will slip by and the pain will start. You may only begin to experience head pain and nausea after the third urination. The moment you realize that a sleep-deprivation migraine has begun, it is time to start working the cure. It is important to note how far the pain has progressed so you will know whether to use the early or full cure, because this headache escalates like lightning. As before, the earlier you begin, the less of a cure you will need.

Regardless of the cure performed, you will need to get some sleep. This is where the cycle comes into focus. The cure will end the pain for some sufferers but not for everyone. Lack of sleep can cause the headache to lock in beyond the ability of the sponge to clean it up, because the lack of sleep is a continuing trigger. This is somewhat like trying to work the dry sponge cure with a bread containing a trigger ingredient such as sunflower seeds.

The only way to approach this headache is to work a combination of the dry sponge cure with much-needed sleep. This will tip the scales in your favor and use your need for sleep as your ally instead of your foe.

1. First you will need to take the acetaminophen, then wait a few minutes to see if you will need the dry sponge.
2. If the pain is abating without sponging your stomach, go on to the next step and get some sleep.
3. If the pain reliever is not reducing the pain enough to help you fall asleep, you will need to dry sponge before you can get some sleep.
4. The last stand is to force yourself to sleep over any residual pain, after you have sponged to the full extent. This may be necessary when the need for sleep maintains the pain lock against all your best efforts. If the pain is still strong enough to make sleep impossible, you will need a sleep aid along with the previous measures.

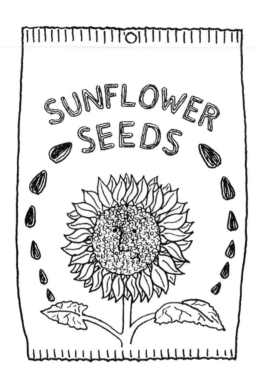

TRIGGER

A NOTE ON SLEEP AIDS: For years all that was available OTC was the same antihistamine (diphenhydramine) used to clear sinuses, re-packaged as a sleeping pill. I found it to be entirely ineffective, although I did breathe better while trying to go to sleep. An irony was occurring in the OTC drug market. A product sold for motion sickness under the brand name Dramamine was more effective for sleeping than the de-congestant sold universally as a sleep aid. This information may come in handy someday when you desperately need sleep and Dramamine is all that is available.

Fortunately, there is finally one OTC product that really works. This is doxylamine succinate, sold under the brand name Unisom and found in most grocery stores. It is a very potent sleep aid. In fact, in my opinion it is almost too potent; I use only one-half the recom-mended dose. Take it after you have worked the cure to the extent that your symptoms warrant and you feel some relief. Sleep will allow the cure to do its full job, while the cure allows sleep. When you awaken, both problems will be solved. The headache will be gone, and a restful sleep will begin a new day.

XV

Migraine Cycles

M igraines appear to occur in a cyclical pattern. This may be a glandularly controlled cycle set to a monthly schedule similar to a menstrual cycle. Many women feel as though these headaches are actually triggered by their menstrual cycles. Although twice as many women as men have migraines, the migraine recurrence cycle seems to function on a monthly schedule with men, just as it does with women.

Regardless of whether you are a man or a woman, mark your calendar after having a migraine, and keep track of your migraine return rate. Also mark your calendar even if you had only an early warning symptom that you treated before a full headache could develop. This will assist you in being extra cautious when the time frame for headache sensitivity approaches.

When the cycle returns, there is a tendency to have migraines in close succession. This is the phenomenon sometimes referred to as "cluster headaches." It seems as though the machinery, once set in motion, easily regains its momentum. The time immediately following a migraine is critical for eating and drinking "tricky," using all the tricks mentioned in this manual.

To put myself out on a limb (and I've been out there so long that I've built a tree house), my belief is that both cycles and clusters are caused by the same stimuli. Our bodies may systematically dump excess gastric juices on a predetermined schedule. My best guess, from out here on my limb, is that the gall bladder dumps cyclically to retain a fresh store of bile. As it empties over two or three days, migraines tend to return or cluster. With women, this occurs in conjunction with the menstrual cycle, while men simply experience it as the gall bladder dump cycle.

XVI

Food Amount Migraines

Two types of migraine are directly related to the amount of food eaten. The first is the *empty-stomach migraine*. Migraine victims run the risk of starting a headache from a lack of regular food intake. This becomes especially troublesome when dieting.

You may have noticed migraine symptoms after prolonged periods without eating. When the stomach has become completely depleted of a nutritional source, in a sense it begins to feed on itself. As the need for nutrition grows and the body is attempting to break down fat cells to obtain energy, extra stomach acid is secreted. When your stomach senses this extra acid secretion, it instantly starts cyclical poisoning. As the headache grows and the stomach locks up, you cease to have hunger pangs as you become overwhelmed by the pain and nausea.

There are three important points to understand about a migraine triggered by hunger. The first is the speed with which it accelerates. Its onset is the most rapid of all migraines, occurring in as little as 15 minutes. An empty stomach allows the migraine to accelerate unimpeded because there is no food to dilute the stomach acid.

The second point is that it's a sure thing. Getting a migraine from hunger is as sure a bet as from eating pizza and a bowl of ice cream before bedtime.

The third and most important point is that eating is absolutely the wrong thing to do if a migraine develops from hunger. Remember, if you get the slightest headache while you're hungry, *do not eat* before working the cure. Eating at this point will trap you into the headache and cause a lengthy cleanup process. On the other hand, if it is treated correctly, this is the easiest migraine to cure because you can use your hunger to rapidly clean out your stomach.

This headache must be treated in two steps:

1. Work the early cure and wait about 10 minutes to see if the pain is diminishing. If it is easing, wait 10 more minutes to feel safely out of danger. If the head pain is leaving and the hunger pangs have returned, or if your stomach is gurgling, indicating that digestion has returned, you have ended your problem. You have opened your stomach and can now eat something non-triggering and drink some orange juice.

2. If you do not feel successful with the early cure, or if you are in any doubt about its effectiveness, simply proceed with the sponging material. I usually sponge before eating anything else, just for insurance.

The other migraine that relates to food amounts is the *overeater's migraine*. This is a condition that takes place when you consistently eat more than your body requires to sustain a healthy, vital, and trim physique. If you are prone to gaining weight and are a migraine sufferer, this condition may play a role in your life.

The physiology of this headache is very simple. As you continue to give your body more nutrition than it needs, it becomes lazy. Just as you become sedate and choose the soft fluff of your couch over the hard surface of a jogging trail, your intestinal tract is having a very similar experience. As your digestive system relaxes, it no longer moves food through at a healthy rate. There is no pressing nutritional need to support aggressive digestion. Under these conditions the slightest provocation will cause the stomach to bottle and start the CAP effect. A normally insignificant amount of any trigger will easily start your migraine.

There are two ways to avoid being susceptible to the overeater's migraine. Naturally, you can cut down on the amount you normally eat ("like, I'm sure you're really gonna do that!"). Or, you can try something you may stand a little better chance of pulling off: start an exercise routine (just walking will help); and get sensible about the blatantly bad stuff you eat.

The role of exercise is so important to a migraine-free life that the following chapter is devoted exclusively to that topic.

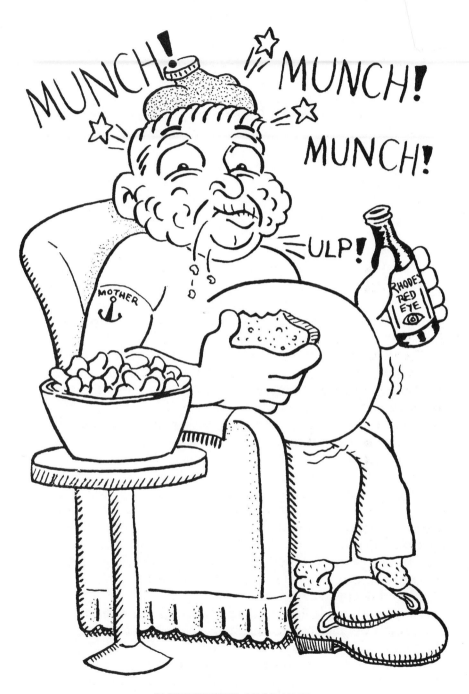

OVEREATER'S MIGRAINE

XVII

Exercise Lifestyle

This is the next-to-last chapter of the manual. I have placed it at the back of the manual so that you would read all of the other advice before reading this. I felt that when I said, "Exercise is more important than the cure," you might not read on. But exercise *is* the single most important component of a migraine-free life. If you follow this advice, the cure will rarely be needed.

The most important and effective lifestyle change you can make is to start a regular exercise program. An intense cardiovascular workout every two or three days, or three times weekly, will virtually end your migraines. Each session should last at least 20 minutes, although an hour is more useful with most exercises. Naturally, this depends entirely on the exercise. You need to use some common sense in determining the amount of time necessary for your workout. If you are speed walking, an hour may be needed; if you are running, a half hour might be all you require. The longer, harder, and more often you exercise, the more you will be insulated from migraines.

Intense full-body and cardiovascular workouts will create a nutritional need in the body that will accelerate the digestive process. Exercise increases the metabolic rate and demands the rapid digestion of food that would otherwise bottle up and become a migraine trigger.

Any form of exercise—such as aerobics, running, speed walking, lap swimming, or bicycling—if done long enough and strong enough, will insulate you from headaches to a 90 percent level. In other words, if you now average 10 migraines in a six-month period, you could

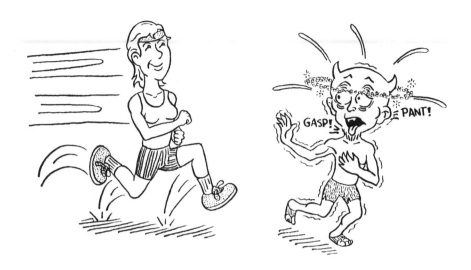

reduce that to one, or none at all. It is important to condition yourself to a consistent exercise routine, because the increase in nutritional need is only effective for about 48 hours.

An exercise program will also pay off in enhanced health and vitality; so get out there and get started. You have nothing to lose, other than a little flab and many potential headaches. On the other hand, you have everything to gain. Exercise is a winning proposition for everyone, but for us migraine sufferers, it's a win-win deal.

XVIII

Looking to the Future

A questionnaire has been inserted in the manual for you to fill out and return to me. I am interested in hearing how your application of the information in this manual has affected your headaches. If you have discovered other foods or procedures that help you, please write and let me know. I will incorporate findings that prove useful into future editions. Hearing from those of you who try this cure is very important. Documentation of the cure's success is essential for future research. Please respond. *Together, we will beat migraines.*

For those of you who are interested, I have formulated an ultra-absorbent muffin for use as a sponging food. The muffin mix is made from a variety of brans, with no fat, as little sugar as is needed to be palatable, and it is prepared in several different flavors. I have added a natural, fruit-based ingredient to stimulate the digestion process and speed the elimination of your migraine. The muffins not only assist in a more rapid cure than the other materials outlined, they are tastier too. If you do want the edge that these muffins offer, you can call the number listed on the order form or simply send it in. The muffins will be shipped to you immediately in a dry mix so that you can have them hot and fresh and save a little on shipping costs.

One last mention. I have made it my life's goal to change the landscape of the migraine world. This may be more than a one-person job. If the lifestyle information and the home cure have worked for you, and if you feel they are important to other migraine sufferers, you can help. There are expenses—such as keeping a database, printing in foreign languages, and extensive advertising—that book sales alone may not cover. Help out only if you see the value in this project. If you do, donations will be kept separate from other income and used solely to accelerate the spread of this information.

For your informational input, monetary donations, or other contributions to this project, thank you.

—Ron Lange

FEEDBACK FORM
(please print)

Last Name _____ First _____ MI ___

Street _____

City _____ State _____ ZIP _____ Phone _____

Sex: F ___ M ___ Age _____ Birthdate _____/_____/ _____ Birthplace _____

Age migraines began _____ Height _____ Weight _____ Chest _____
(Measure chest in inches at solar plexus under pectoral major muscle. Women—do not include breasts.)

Describe your success with MASTER YOUR MIGRAINE general info: _____

_____

_____

Describe your success with the DRY STOMACH SPONGE:_____

_____

_____

Have you tried Migraine Muffins? _____ How well did they work? _____

What sponging materials have you tried other than what is in the book, and how well have they worked?

_____

_____

_____

Describe your headaches: _____

_____

_____

How long do they last, how frequent are they, and is there a cycle of frequency (i.e., monthly)?

_____

_____

Describe the extent of your nausea in terms of frequency and duration: _____

_____

If you drink, how much weekly? _____ If you smoke, how much daily? _____

List any personal triggers not mentioned in the book: _____

_____

List medications you have taken for migraines in the past and their effect: _____

_____

What new OTC pain relievers have you used, and what weight-to-dosage amount succeeded in opening your stomach? _____

_____

_____

List family members (by relation) who suffer from migraines: _____

_____

_____

Use top ⅓ of back side for additional info. Fold as indicated, tape closed, put on stamp, and mail back. Thank you for responding.